What professionals are saying about this book!

Women will be smiling and nodding in recognition of themselves on each page. As is well stated within the book, "Life is too short to stuff a mushroom." This and other one-liners will be quickly adopted by women with AD/HD across the globe.—*Wilma Fellman, M.Ed., LPC, author of "The Other Me", and "Finding A Career That Works for You." Contributing author of "Understanding Women with AD/HD"*

Anyone who has ever felt stuck or overwhelmed by life's demands will appreciate the fun, humor and practical tips to be found in the pages of *Survival Tips for Women with AD/HD*. Buy this book and keep it handy for those inevitable times when you are standing around asking yourself "what do I do now?"—*Kate Kelly, MSN, ACT, co-author of "You Mean I'm Not Lazy, Stupid or Crazy?!" and "The ADDed Dimension." Founder of The ADDed Dimension Coaching Group. ADD coach in private practice.*

Kudos to this multitalented woman for writing an easy to read book that is both poignant and pragmatic. I laughed and cried, and most important, I learned many new strategies for managing my AD/HD.—*Linda Halperin, Ed.S. School Psychologist*

Survival Tips for Women with AD/HD is for us, women who have AD/HD, and is written...with great heart and hope and large helpings of practical common sense. Five gold stars out of five to Ms. Matlen for her A+ book.—*Christine A. Adamec, Author of "Moms with ADD: A Self-Help Manual"*

Survival Tips for Women with AD/HD: Beyond Piles, Palms & Post-its

by Terry Matlen, M.S.W.

Illustrations by Peter Welleman

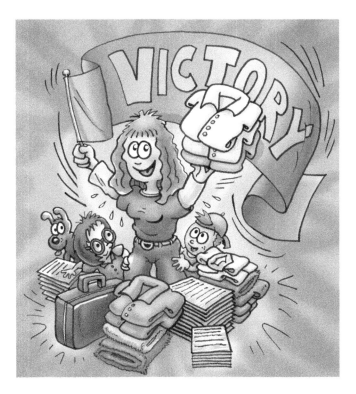

Specialty Press, Inc.
300 N.W. 70th Ave.
Plantation, Florida 33317

Library of Congress Cataloging-in-Publication Data

Matlen, Terry, 1953-
    Survival tips for women with AD/HD: beyond piles, palms & post-its/ by Terry Matlen.
        p. cm.
    ISBN 1-886941-59-9 (alk. paper)
    1. Attention-deficit disorder in adults—Popular works. 2. Attention-deficit-disordered adults—Life skills guides. 3. Mothers—Life skills guides. 4. Women—Life skills guides. 5. Time management. 6. Scheduling. I. Title.

RC394.A85M36 2005
616.85'89'0082—dc22
                                                          2004059036
ISBN 1-886941-59-9

Illustrations by Peter Welleman
Cover Design by Michael Kall

10 9 8 7 6 5 4 3

Printed in the United States of America
Specialty Press, Inc.
300 Northwest 70th Avenue, Suite 102
Plantation, Florida 33317
(954) 792-8100 • (800) 233-9273
www.addwarehouse.com

Dedication

First and foremost, this book is dedicated to my family: Jerry, Kate, and Mackenzie, who are the love of my life. It is also dedicated to my mother, Helen Wachler, who gave me—and continues to give me—the courage to follow my dreams. And to women with AD/HD worldwide who live with determination and hope, waiting for the world to catch up with them.

Table of Contents

Page

Foreword by Sari Solden, M.S., LMFT   vii
Acknowledgements   xiii
Preface   xvii

Chapters
1   From Me to You: Validating Your Experiences   1
2   Carry That Weight: What You Don't Know
    Can Hurt You   7
3   Here, There, and Everywhere: Specifics
    of Organizing Your House   15
       Organizing the Kitchen   15
       Closets, Shelves, and All the
          Stuff Inside!   19
       Kids and Their Clutter   20
       Paper   21
       Organizing in General   26
4   Strawberry Fields: Meals and Entertaining   29
       Grocery Shopping   29
       Cooking   32
       Meal Planning   37
       Entertaining   43
5   Fixing a Hole: How to Delegate, Eliminate, and
    Simplify Household Chores   47
       Laundry   47
       Cleaning and Decluttering   51
       Dishes   54
       Errands   56
       Miscellaneous Chores   57

Table of Contents

6	She's a Woman: Personal Tips on Clothes Shopping, Health, Hypersensitivities, and Leisure Time	61
	Clothes: Shopping and Dressing	62
	Health	65
	Hypersensitivities	67
	Sleep	73
	Miscellaneous	74
	Travel	75
	Leisure Time	76
	Setting Goals and Completing Projects	77
7	I Should Have Known Better: School and Studying	81
	Study Strategies	81
	Academic Difficulties	83
8	A Hard Day's Night: Thriving on the Job	87
	Careers	87
	Reminders	89
	Organizing Taks	90
	Minimizing Distractions	91
	Scheduling	93
	Clutter	94
	General Tips	94
9	Any Time at All: Time and Data Management	97
	Data Management	98
	Planners	99
	Capturing Ideas	101
	Timers	104
	General Time Management Advice	105
10	We Can Work it Out: Relationships and Social Skills	111
	General Advice	111
	Support	112
	Communication Skills	113

11	Come Together: Parenting and Family	119
	Behavior and Discipline	119
	Traveling with Kids	123
	Sleep	124
	Minimizing Distractions	124
	Chores	126
	Balancing Family Time with Self-regeneration	127
	Connecting	127
12	Money: Managing Finances	135
	Paying Bills	136
	Saving Money	139
13	I've Just Seen a Face (But I Can't for the Life of Me Remember the Name): Memory Tips	143
	Capturing Ideas	143
	Keeping Track of Things	145
	Physiology of Memory	146
	Miscellaneous Memory Tips	147
	Math	148
	Names	149
	Directions	150
	Reminders	151
	Timers	152
14	Revolution: Technology	155
	Creative ways to Use a Palm Pilot	155
	Internet, Computers, and Cell Phones	159
15	With a Little Help from My Friends: Humor for the Soul	163
	You Know You Have AD/HD When...	163
	Stories to Tickle the Funny Bone	176
	Kitchen Chaos	178
	10 Things to Never Do in the Kitchen (with no appologies to David Letterman)	180
	Quotes from the Impatient Patients	183
16	Help: Tips from Coaches and Professional Organizers	193

	Tips from Professional Coaches	193
	Tips from Professional Organizers	211
17	...Speaking Words of Wisdom: Top AD/HD Experts Share Their Stories	225
18	Savoy Truffle: SOS Recipes	255
19	Do You Want to Know a Secret? Books, Tapes, Web sites, Newsletters, and More	287
	Books and Video Tapes	287
	Media: Web sites, Newsletters, Mailing Lists Magazines, and Catalogs	294
	Support	299
	Products	304
References		321
Appendix		323
	Month-of-Meals System	324
	How to Keep a Kitchen Clean	325
	Prioritizing Chart	327
	Affirmation List	328
	Record Your Own Tips	329
Index		333

Foreword

by Sari Solden, M.S, LMFT

I have known Terry professionally since 1995 when my book *Women with Attention Deficit Disorder* was first published. At that time, Terry was just starting to become involved in the field of women with AD/HD and was seeking some guidance. I was proud to mentor her and watched as she steadily assumed positions of increasing influence in the field. In the years since, I have witnessed her work tirelessly and with great devotion to enable countless isolated women to survive and thrive in a non-AD/HD world by connecting them with others and often difficult to find services.

Terry has a true gift for bringing people together in a variety of creative ways such as newsletters, online conferences, coaching and support groups so that they can learn from one another and share insights. She has steadily built a powerful network of professionals, adults, and parents both locally and globally. On several occasions, people from around the world have written me long, detailed, heartbreaking messages with pleas for specialized kinds of help such as, "I need an expert in women with AD/HD in Alaska," or "I need a doctor for medication in Japan," or "Can you find me a good therapist in a small town in Iowa?" What a relief it was to have someone like Terry to refer them to for help. With her combination of a caring nature, talent for tracking down the right resources, and creativity, Terry has always been able to find a solution or a new approach to the problem.

Many years ago when the Internet was just getting popular, she was one of the first to offer online support groups for women with AD/HD. I still remember that remarkable moment at a national Attention Deficit Disorder Association (ADDA) conference when several of these women who had been meeting online from all over the globe for so long finally came together for the first time in person. There were hugs and tears, but mostly I remember the laughter—starting from the moment they met and continuing for the rest of the several days they spent together. It had a kind of "separated at birth" feeling—they were *home* again with people for whom they felt an intense kinship and identification. Many of them forged strong bonds that still continue today and many still meet each year at the annual conference.

In addition to her online support groups, Terry has deepened and broadened her involvement in the field of AD/HD by taking on increasingly active roles in groups such as *Children and Adults with Attention Deficit Disorder* (CHADD) and the *Attention Deficit Disorder Association* (ADDA). She has gathered resources and mobilized people to expand and improve CHADD's support network here in Michigan and has worked on the ADDA board for many years to develop high-quality conferences all across the country. She has also been an unflagging advocate for those with AD/HD, answering media questions and fighting stereotypes in order to improve the public's understanding of AD/HD.

Terry has also developed a solid reputation as a presenter at local and national conferences. As a result of her numerous contacts over the years with both professionals and clients, she is able to draw on her extensive knowledge base regarding AD/HD issues to infuse her presentations with wisdom, information, and support, offering titles such as "Chaos in the Kitchen," "Survival Tips for Women with AD/HD," and "Parenting with Distractions: Surviving Family Life when You AND Your Child Have AD/HD."

Now, in this book, Terry uses her ability to gather people and resources to extend what she has been doing online, at conferences, and in her practice all these years—connecting people who are isolated and letting them "talk" to each other, giving them a voice and a place to share all the strategies and wisdom they have gathered. This book gives women with AD/HD the chance to hear from other women like themselves *in their own words*, how they have confronted and coped with many of the same specific struggles. Because of this, Terry's book may have a dramatic and validating effect on women with AD/HD by making it clear to them that they are not alone. The most commonly reported benefit for readers of *Women with Attention Deficit Disorder,* has been the great sense of relief and validation they feel when they realize that other women experience their same challenges. Reading *Survival Tips for Women* is like attending one big support group with Terry!

And because the tips in this book have been written by women who actually experience these difficulties and have found their own solutions, the suggestions make more sense to those with AD/HD than do some of the approaches designed by others who don't understand the complexity and the real feel from the inside. Since this book focuses on women's issues and the challenges they face as their day-to-day tasks collide with the realities of their AD/HD, it can help women reduce and defuse some of the shame, guilt, and frustration that often accompany these problems.

Terry's warmth, humor, knowledge, and empathy have always shone through in her writings and presentations—this book is no exception. She writes openly and expressively about her own journey, providing the reader with stories that are both instructive and inspirational. Terry's friendly, highly personal, readable style leaves readers feeling as if Terry is speaking directly to them. Terry knows about AD/HD in women deeply and thoroughly—as a women with ADD, as a mother, as a professional, and as an expert in the field—she is the real deal.

As the sub-title "Beyond Piles, Palms & Post-its" suggests, the book gives survival tips and much more. Terry understands that the keys for women to live successfully with AD/HD are self-acceptance, learning to get support from others, and focusing on one's strengths. *Survival Tips for Women with AD/HD* provides a wealth of tips and strategies, but readers will also absorb the important underlying message that even if they never master these kinds of tasks, they can still thrive. They can still be mature, responsible, warm, caring, competent women—these difficulties *do* not and *can* not define them—unless they let them!

In this way, the book is healing, as well as practical. This is what separates it from other functional guides. Terry has also asked AD/HD professionals to contribute their struggles and triumphs, not from a professional view point alone, but from the heart about what has made the difference for them in their own lives. This book may look like a simple collection of tips, but it is thoughtful additions like these that help it go to the core of what women with AD/HD need to hear.

Like an emergency tool kit, every woman with AD/HD should have this book. A reader can pick it up when no ideas are occurring to her, too many are flooding in, or when she feels stuck, overwhelmed, or ready to shut down. She can just reach for this book and feel reassured and relaxed enough to be able to figure out a new way to proceed. For Terry's reader, this book is like being at a gathering of women who really get AD/HD, get her, and know what her life is like.

Women, when you are overwhelmed, panicked at the thought of what to make for dinner, how to deal with unexpected guests, or any of the many other secret struggles in the lives of women with AD/HD, you can reach for this book and find a wise and warm guide in Terry. Anytime you need an understanding friend, just open to any page and you are likely to find the kind of help and support you need from all the women who are speaking directly to you in Survival Tips for Women with AD/HD.

Sari Solden, M.S, LMFT
Author of *Women with Attention Deficit Disorder*
and *Journeys through ADDulthood*
Ann Arbor, MI
www.sarisolden.com

Acknowledgements

My deepest thanks go to the hundreds of AD/HD women who participated in this project. This book would not have been possible without their generous gifts of time and effort.

In fact, *Survival Tips* would never have seen the light of day had it not been for the many friends, family, and colleagues who supported me through the ups and downs of seeing this project come to life. To that end, I would like to first thank my editor, Jeanne Ballew, who early on recognized my strengths and weaknesses and supported them both. Her astute eye and gentle coaching kept me going, always keeping me on track.

Special thanks go to Dr. Harvey Parker of Specialty Press for believing in me and this project enough to give "voice" to my ideas and reality to my dreams through the vehicle of this book.

Thanks to Tara McGillicuddy for helping me solicit and organize tips from the many AD/HD women online. Without her help, I would have floundered in a sea of emails.

To Dan Connaghan, my masterful web wizard, I thank him for recreating a bigger and better ADDConsults.com. His incredible skills, reliability, and generosity of time have been so appreciated.

I would like to thank my colleagues, many of whom have also become friends, for their support, feedback, and personal involvement in this book: Kate Kelly, R.N., M.S.N., Dr. Ned Hallowell, Thom Hartmann, Dr. Patricia Quinn, Dr.

Russell Barkley, Dr. Lynn Weiss, Dr. Peter Jaksa, Dr. Michele Novotni, Nancy Ratey, Ed.M., MCC, David Giwerc, MCC, ICF, Dr. Arthur Robin, Dr. John Bailey, Mary Jane Johnson, PCC, ACT, Linda Anderson, M.A., MCC, and Kerch McConlogue, CPCC.

Thanks to Dr. Robert Underhill for his wisdom and kindness. And yes, I will continue to paint!

Thanks to Sari Solden, M.S., LMFT, pioneer and mentor, for her guidance and encouragement. She has truly been an inspiration to me, both professionally and personally. Without her contributions to the field of women and AD/HD, I, along with countless others, would never have been able to find the missing piece that explains my quirks, foibles, and challenges. I know I speak for many when I thank her from the bottom of my heart.

Many thanks to my friends Eleanor Payson, M.S.W. and Dr. Sally Palaian whose own literary dreams helped to spur mine.

To my friends Deborah Lancaster, Becky Booth, Sue Barringer, Corine Schramke, Suzanne Howe, Linda O'Brien, and Shannon Taylor—I thank them for always being there for me, online or in person.

Special thanks to Linda Halperin, MA, Ed.S., who pulled me into the ADDA world headfirst and who has been a constant source of strength.

To Jeri Goldstein, MC, APRN, who burns the midnight oil with me while discussing the meaning of life, art, and psychology.

I'd also like to thank my dear friend and colleague, Wilma Fellman, M.Ed., LPC, whose daily dash of humor, optimism, and eternal wisdom have helped me stay steady, not only in this book project, but in life in general. I have learned a lot by observing her positive spirit.

To Lila Kadaj, my dearest sister-friend who shares this journey with me. She has always been an inspiration to me, co-exploring the many avenues of creative and intellectual enlightenment. She will be my soul sister through life!

I would like to remember and honor my beloved grandmother, Mollie Zolkower, who taught me to love the human spirit and who delighted in being with people by finding the best in them. I will always miss you.

To my step-dad Norman Wachler, who is my real dad in spirit, for he has always been there for me in his quiet, loving way.

There aren't words to express what the love and strength of a mother can do for a timid, fearful child who then grows up to be a confident woman with children of her own. Special thanks to my mother, Helen Wachler, for believing in me, cheering me on through thick and thin, and always being there for me even during those early years of turbulence. She has been my confidante, my inspiration...and my fashion advisor. She has taught me more than she'll ever know, and though I may have inherited her entrepreneurial and creative ways, I missed out somehow on the cooking and dancing genes. I will always be grateful for her support of my endless projects ...and for never asking me to bring a dish that requires more than two ingredients! Thanks to her, too, for killing all of those spiders in my bedroom and for checking under the bed for that scary madman in hiding, waiting to grab my ankles.

I would like to thank my daughters, Kate and Mackenzie, for putting up with "Cousin It" who has replaced their mom this past year since they mainly saw the back of my head while working on this book.

To Kate, I love her more than words can say. Her kindness, intelligence, talents, and beauty have awed and inspired me. I am so utterly proud of her.

To Mackenzie, whose challenges led me to learn about my own, I love her for her upbeat spirit, good humor, and caring ways. I am so proud to be her mom!

They say that a healthy marriage can only occur when the effort is 50/50, but in my case, my dearest husband, Jerry, has given way more than his share this past year as I worked on this book. Thanks to him for his never failing love, support, and belief in me and for keeping me laughing even after 25 years together. How I appreciate him for never complaining about mystery dinners or late night runs for carry-out! But most of all, I thank him for working so hard to keep our love alive.

Many thanks to you all!

Terry Matlen

September, 2004

Preface

*Success is achieved when you figure out what you were born
to do and fashion a lifestyle that enables you to do it (p. 404).*
Kate Kelly and Peggy Ramundo
You Mean I'm Not Lazy, Stupid or Crazy?!

After a day at the supermarket with her two children in tow
and a third in a baby carrier, a woman we'll call Karen se-
curely fastened her children into her grocery-filled car and
pulled out of the parking lot. Pedestrians gaped at the driver,
hands frantically pointing to the top of the car. Puzzled, Karen
stopped the car to see what the fuss was about. She was absolutely horrified to realize that she'd left the baby carrier—
and the baby—sitting on the roof of her car. Luckily, she
retrieved her youngest and settled him in the backseat of her
car thereby averting what would have been a horrible trag-
edy.

Fortunately, most women with AD/HD don't do things
this extreme—but most any of them will tell you that it is not
so far-fetched that they couldn't imagine themselves doing
something like this. Let's put it this way—it's on the con-
tinuum.

According to the prestigious Mayo Clinic, it is estimated
that 7.5% of school-aged children have AD/HD. More than
70% of these children grow up to be adults with AD/HD. In

other words, there are between 4.5 to 5.5 *million* women in the US alone with AD/HD (Barbaresi et al., 2002; R. Barkley, personal communication, August 18, 2004).

Unfortunately, the great majority of these women have not been diagnosed or treated for their AD/HD. Perhaps if Karen's AD/HD had been appropriately addressed, the vignette above might never have occurred. Tormented by the daily chores and decisions needed to survive in a world of linear thinkers, millions of AD/HD women find themselves drowning in the chaos of their non-linear lives. Post-its and Palm Pilots serve as their daily life preservers—*if* they are lucky enough to know how to use them. What comes so easily to most such as organizing papers, paying bills, cooking the family dinner, and getting to work on time can be beyond the scope of possibility for the woman with AD/HD.

I am one of those women. I have never left one of my kids on the roof of my car or forgotten them at a shopping mall. But like you, I have—and still do—struggle with heaps of laundry, meal preparations that cause more anxiety than gastronomic bliss, and relentless piles of papers.

Let me share with you some of my own personal and professional journeys that may shed some light on what motivated me to put this book together. For years I struggled with significant anxiety symptoms and was treated with medication and therapy. I'm certain I was born anxious, or at the very least, was wired to become anxious when all the environmental pieces merged with my neurological predisposition. Along with therapy and anxiety medication, exercise and meditation also helped alleviate some of the symptoms, but I still felt something was "off." Anxiety couldn't explain why I was unable to talk to someone if there was the slightest noise in the background. I shunned phone conversations because I needed to "see" the person's mouth moving in order to stay connected. Worse, if there was a TV on even in the farthest room in the house, I couldn't hear a thing the person on the phone was saying!

I did earn two college degrees, both in subjects dear to my heart: a B.S. in Art Education in 1975 and a M.S.W. in Clinical Social Work in 1979. As a student, I suffered with a poor self-image, figuring it was just a fluke that I'd done so well in college (it wasn't till much later that I learned that if I focused on subjects that were of interest to me, I could do exceptionally well). Luckily, I made some good vocational choices, though I learned in my last semester of art education studies that I wasn't cut out to be a teacher; I simply couldn't handle the chaos of a classroom. That led to two years of fine arts courses in painting, until I realized that only a handful of painters in this country actually made a living unless they were willing to work three additional jobs. In the end, my insatiable interest in psychology led me to enter the social work program.

Before having children, I worked with severely mentally ill adolescents in an outpatient mental health clinic. In those days, I struggled with the overwhelming amount of paperwork but figured that was just a personality "fluke." After all, I was never able to keep my bedroom in order as a kid, why would my office be any different? So I plugged along, doing my best, making sure the piles were hidden in drawers and filing cabinets at the end of the day.

I left my job when my daughter Kate was born in 1985; Mackenzie followed soon after in 1988. At first, I was thrilled that life would be easier without deadlines or masses of paperwork to contend with and knowing that I could focus all of my energy on doing what I had yearned to do my whole life: being a parent. But I was in for a huge surprise—my life was about to get more complicated than I'd ever dreamed possible. Even though I had a post-graduate college degree,

I was incapable of remembering to do the family laundry. Papers were in piles everywhere, and bills were often paid late. What was wrong with me??

In terms of AD/HD, I hit the wall when I turned 36 in 1989. Of course, I had no idea at the time that I was struggling with AD/HD. All I knew was that I couldn't handle the bustling household that contained two very hyperactive and impulsive children. Finally, after a particularly stressful phone conversation in which I was unable to hear my husband on the other end while the children were playing relatively quietly at my feet, I wondered if my problems could be due to a hearing loss. Excited, I made an appointment to see if that could be the cause of my "phone frustrations" and also my inability to follow conversations in groups, but I was shocked to find that my hearing was actually better than average.

At around the same time, my then 16-month-old daughter, Mackenzie, became perilously ill with encephalitis following a routine infant vaccination. Luckily she survived the insult but not without significant residual damage. Since this disease affects the lining of the brain, one of the outcomes of that devastating illness was that she developed what is known as "acquired AD/HD," which means she wasn't born with AD/HD but developed it due to the brain injury. Along with the AD/AD, she also became mildly cognitively impaired and still struggles with speech and language disorders, learning disabilities, and more.

While learning how to help her with her severe hyperactivity, impulsivity, and distractibility (this is a child who literally *did* bounce off the walls), I began to read articles and books on AD/HD. For some reason still unknown to me, I also picked up a book on adult AD/HD, and a light bulb went off in my head. I recognized several family members in the description of how AD/HD presents in adults, and as I continued to do more research, I had another epiphany while reading about the inattentive AD/HD subtype. My journey had begun. I went for an evaluation and was formally diagnosed with AD/HD.

Because of the many years of treatment for my anxiety, I went through quite a long period of denial about AD/HD. In the book, *Women with Attention Deficit Disorder*, Sari Solden discusses the phases many, if not all, women go though when first diagnosed with AD/HD. For me, the denial consumed me. But finally, I was able to move on and get the appropriate treatment and support for it. After a number of years, I was finally able to reframe what I long had thought were character weaknesses as symptoms of AD/HD and learned how to break through the many roadblocks that had compromised my self-esteem.

On a professional level, I can only say that the impact of learning about AD/HD was utterly transformational. When I learned how treatable this condition was and how my own treatment had affected my life in such a positive way, I decided to take my mission "on the road" and help other women with AD/HD. If I could become productive and successful despite my own AD/HD, I knew others could as well.

I started my private practice in 1995, offering psychotherapy solely to AD/HD adults, and a few years later, expanded my practice to include AD/HD coaching, as well. After a number of years, it became evident that the needs of my youngest daughter required that I work at home, so in 2000 I launched ADD Consults (www.addconsults.com), an online AD/HD clinic that offers consultations, online conferences, a store, articles, a professional and coach directory, and other online resources for anyone with Internet access. There are support groups available on my website for men and women, with one group offered weekly for women only, in which they can share their triumphs and frustrations while garnering and sharing support to all who visit the chat room. My motivation for offering these support chats was born from my own experience early on in my own AD/HD journey, when I would attend similar chats on AOL, then later would moderate and co-lead groups for women. I knew firsthand how helpful it was to connect with other AD/HD women.

In 1994, in an effort to further expand my knowledge and networks to better assist myself, my family, and my clients, I began attending our local CHADD (Children and Adults with AD/HD) chapter religiously until I decided it was time for me to give back in a measurable way. As a result, I served as the coordinator from 1996 to 2002, formed its first support group for AD/HD adults, and began attending its annual conferences. My involvement with CHADD spurred me on to attend ADDA's (Attention Deficit Disorder Association) first national conference; their focus is more on the needs of adults with AD/HD. Going to ADDA, meeting the top AD/HD experts in the world, and connecting with hundreds of adults who also had AD/HD was a life altering experience for me. I was so excited by what this group was doing that soon after, in 1998, I joined ADDA's board of directors and subsequently served as vice-president from 2000 until 2003; I still remain on the board today. And in order to develop and maintain my local connections, I joined MAAAN (Michigan Adolescent/Adult ADD Network for Professionals), serve on my local school district's Parent Advisory Committee, and am a board member of our district's Friends of Different Learners, a parent advocacy group. In addition, I have presented at local and national conferences ranging from Seattle to Norfolk (including CHADD and ADDA) and continue to do so approximately five to six times a year. I've been interviewed numerous times on radio and by newspapers and magazines and was invited to participate in the "AD/HD Experts On Call Annual Call-in" in New York City. These wonderful opportunities have been extremely gratifying, empowering and enriching. I strongly encourage each and every one of you to seek out such groups and get involved. Not that you have to make learning about AD/HD your life, but the more you know and the more support you can find, the more empowered you will be.

You could say that sharing information on AD/HD is my calling. To that end, I've written numerous articles for publications such as FOCUS, (a newsletter published by ADDA), ADDitude Magazine, ADDvance, etc. and for many Web sites, including my own. The Internet has been a tremendous vehicle for connecting with those with AD/HD. In addition to my chat room, I developed and continue to moderate an AD/HD Professionals online mailing list to promote awareness and information for professionals, which has over 300 members worldwide.

Add to all of these various roles the fact that I am also an accomplished oil painter (Yes, I hung on to that dream!) who has had work displayed in galleries and shows both nationally and locally (including a major museum), for over thirty years, and am also a musician who plays acoustic guitar, piano, drums, and bass. My intent in sharing all of these accomplishments is not to toot my own horn but to give you a sense of what can be accomplished despite having AD/HD. Yes, I still struggle on a daily basis, and sometimes I bite off more than I can chew but with the support of those around me, the benefits I've gained from receiving appropriate treatment, the help I've gotten by learning to ask, and the self-acceptance I've gained from changing my expectations for myself, I've been able to thrive and take steps to fulfill my purpose here. You can do the same.

Terry Matlen, M.S.W., A.C.S.W.
www.addconsults.com

Chapter 1

From Me to You:
Validating Your Experiences

In the ten years or so that I've been talking to adults who have AD/HD, I've been listening intently to their struggles, noting their solutions, and collecting their insights. When I decided to share this wisdom with others through the vehicle of this book, I sent word out via email announcements, my newsletter, my presentations, and word of mouth that I was looking for tips from women with AD/HD. They were invited to email me or fill out a form on either my Web site or my colleague Tara McGillicuddy's Web site and hundreds of tips came rolling in. (Please note that only the first name, last initial, and location were used for those who sent in a tip but didn't respond to my request for permission to edit their submissions. Only the first name and last initial were used for those who failed to respond to my request for additional information such as location.)

By compiling years of accumulated knowledge from my clients, women all over the world, and top AD/HD experts in the field who have found ways to live successfully with, or in spite of, their AD/HD, I hope to encourage other women with AD/HD like you to find happiness and success in your lives. There is nothing more empowering than knowing that you aren't alone in your struggles. In *Survival Tips for Women with AD/HD*, you will experience a powerful connection with women worldwide who share the very same trials.

Many adults with AD/HD have lived for years in shame, depressed that they can't do what for others seem to be such simple things. This book fills the void by offering pragmatic, concrete solutions to daily problems, submitted by women with AD/HD *for* other women with AD/HD. With a dash of humor and an artillery of weapons to accomplish your goals in bold, creative ways, you can now move forward with confidence. You will become more capable as a mother, spouse, daughter, friend, co-worker, student, and more. You can reach your fullest potential, both personally and professionally, by becoming more efficient and productive. As AD/HD expert, Dr. Ned Hallowell says in his book *Driven to Distraction*, "ADD adults need lots of encouragement. This is in part due to many self-doubts that have accumulated over the years….[they] whither without encouragement and thrive when given it" (Hallowell & Ratey, 1994, p. 246).

Reading these tips from fellow women with AD/HD will not only offer real tools for living that can boost your confidence but will also relieve the guilt and anxiety so many have when they feel they don't measure up to the norms of today's society—the woman who can—and *should*—"do it all!" These proven gems will help you get through the piles of laundry on your floor to the piles of paper on your desk with a feeling of accomplishment, knowing that you fought the good fight.

A common complaint from women with AD/HD has been that husbands, parents, siblings, friends, bosses, etc. don't believe that they truly struggle or that their challenges are authentic. If they only tried "harder," they could *do it*. As the emails started pouring in, it dawned on me that with this book, women with AD/HD could now proclaim that they are not the only ones who labor over seemingly simple tasks. *Survival Tips for Women with AD/HD* is proof, validation, that others are similarly challenged *and* have found solutions. Like the well-titled book by Kate Kelly and Peggy Ramundo, *You Mean I'm Not Lazy, Stupid or Crazy?!*, we are not any of these but rather women whose neurology sometimes gets in the way of our daily lives.

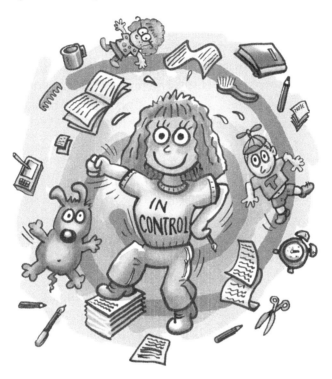

Survival Tips for Women with AD/HD is your manual, your guide. There's no need to read it cover to cover; just look up your trouble spots in the index as they come up and see how others have handled similar roadblocks. By the way, you may be wondering why I chose Beatles' titles for the chapters in this book. They symbolize for me my own struggles during a turbulent adolescence when my deep loneliness, anxiety, and pain were brightened and relieved by listening to—and learning to play—Beatles' songs. While other teenagers were out socializing, I spent most of my after school hours as a loner, playing guitar and learning songs to ease the hurt of not fitting in. The titles remind me of where I was then and how far I've come—it truly is a "Long and Winding Road."

The next chapter is an introduction to some of the symptoms of AD/HD that you won't hear from your doctor, as well as a deeper dive into how such symptoms can impact the lives of women with AD/HD and those they love. The following chapters present survival tips from many women with AD/HD around the world and cover a range of advice on how to deal with issues such as the following:

- Paperwork at home and at the office
- Planning and executing meals
- Social situations and relationship skills
- Paying bills on time
- Organizing and cleaning the house
- Clothes shopping and wardrobe advice
- Health
- Memory jogs

The final chapters offer humorous anecdotes, tips from professional coaches and organizers, personal insights from AD/HD experts, and a list of ADD-friendly recipes, as well as a comprehensive resource list of books, Web sites, newsletters, and more.

By the time that you've picked up this book, chances are that you have already been diagnosed with AD/HD and are on a treatment plan. Although this book is geared for women like you, it may also be helpful to any harried woman living in the twenty-first century, including the following:

- Stay at home mothers
- Working mothers

4

- Single mothers
- Executive women
- Creative, non-linear thinking women

I invite you to share the journeys of these creative, bright women, note what has worked for them and to try out some— or many—of their ideas yourself. Use the worksheet at the back of the book to add some tips of your own to refer back to or please send your tips to my Web form at: www.addconsults.com/book.php for a possible second edition to this book.

One thing I routinely remind my clients of is that although AD/HD can interfere with daily living in a big way, it isn't a death sentence. Learning coping mechanisms and strategies can take you far in your journey from just surviving to embracing it, as Sari Solden describes it in *Women with Attention Deficit Disorder* (1995):

> Embracing all of what you are is one of the important keys to heal self-esteem wounds, to improve your mood by improving your self-talk, and to give you a strong sense of an inner core that doesn't reel from shame when ADD symptoms still inevitably occur. Embracing helps you move through the "grief cycle" to a deep sense of acceptance and *beyond*, to actual *enjoyment* of your ADD and your creativity. (p. 205)

Celebrate your differences, for you truly are unique. Keep in mind, too, some of the lighter sides of living and coping with AD/HD. As one woman with AD/HD says, "It's like carrying around a 24-hour party in my brain!" When you're having your own AD/HD moment, instead of agoniz-

5

ing over what you did wrong, remind yourself that it's just your AD/HD kicking in. As my husband is fond of saying, I make the only roast that tastes like sliced wallet. Years ago that would have crushed my then fragile self-esteem. Now, it has become a family joke. You may not be the world's best chef, but maybe you are a gifted poet, a loyal friend, or a creative artist. Though research studies haven't yet proven this, I've found in my own clinical work with women with AD/HD, that they tend to be the most sensitive, creative, warm, and funny people I've ever met. So don't compromise your core being. As Judy Garland once said, "Always be a first-rate version of yourself instead of a second-rate version of somebody else."

Chapter 2

Carry that Weight: What You Don't Know Can Hurt You

By the time that you've discovered this book, you've learned that AD/HD does indeed exist and that it's not only about little boys in school who can't sit still and who throw spit balls behind the teacher's back. You may know now that your daily duels with paper piles, "creative" time management, agonizing social faux pas, and inconsistent attention are not weaknesses, personality flaws, or the result of poor parenting. Perhaps you've gone to a mental health specialist and have been officially diagnosed with AD/HD. You now have a working definition of it, a fairly good understanding of the cause and effect, and a course of treatment that often involves a combination of the following: counseling, medication, support such as AD/HD coaching, and education. If you're really gung ho, you've read some of the more popular books on AD/HD on how to organize your life in ten easy steps. The books are great—but still…something is missing from your "toolbox"—something that explains all your little quirks and foibles, but more importantly, the differences you've felt your whole life.

Have you wondered all these years if you are the only one on the planet who faces these situations?

- Why can I see your mouth moving but can't hear any words?
- Why do I have panic attacks in the mall?
- Why does my skin crawl when I am touched in certain ways?
- Why does the thought of going to Disneyworld make me feel nauseated instead of excited like everybody else?
- Why am I unable to put together a single outfit when I look through my closet filled with blouses and skirts?
- Why can I obtain a college degree yet can't

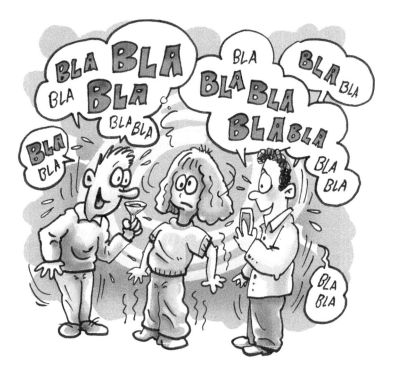

figure out what to cook every night let alone remember to get the ingredients while at the grocery store?

- Why, in social groups, am I unable to get the words out that are floating around in my head?
- Why does the sight of a pile of dirty laundry make my heart palpitate?

The core symptoms of AD/HD described in clinical journals and books include inattention, impulsivity, and hyperactivity. Another symptom of AD/HD often seen in both men and women is disorganization. This is one that helps explain why women with AD/HD struggle with seemingly simple tasks such as picking out clothes, keeping their home in order, handling paperwork at their jobs, etc.

Being a woman with AD/HD can cause impairment in many areas of one's daily life. This can be due to the core symptoms of AD/HD *and* the effects of associated conditions (anxiety, depression, learning problems, etc.) that are often found in people with AD/HD. Take a look at the many ways this can impact your life:

- Low self-worth
- Easily overwhelmed
- Hypersensitive to criticism
- Emotionally charged; easily upset
- Irritable
- Tendency to ruminate
- Poor sense of time; often run late
- Start projects but can't seem to finish them
- Take on too much both personally and professionally
- Difficulty making decisions
- Get confused when more than one person is talking
- Can't filter out sounds

- Need extra time to process what is being said
- Can't remember the theme of a movie within minutes of leaving the theatre
- Forget the details of a book you just read
- Splintered skills: brilliant in some areas but severely challenged in others
- Poor sense of direction; can't read maps or blueprints
- Struggle to visualize things (out of sight, out of mind)
- Difficulty remembering names
- Say things without thinking, often hurting others' feelings
- Appear self-absorbed
- Don't seem to hear what others are saying
- Talk too much
- Talk too little; can't figure out how to enter a discussion
- Don't "get" jokes
- Can't say "no"
- Hypersensitive to noise, touch, smell
- Clumsy with poor coordination; always bumping into things
- Difficulty falling asleep and difficulty waking up the next morning
- Tire easily, or, conversely, can't sit still
- Experience severe PMS
- Poor math and/or writing skills
- Problem with word retrieval
- Poor handwriting
- Have difficulty with boring, repetitive tasks
- Difficulty with self-control in areas such as shopping, eating, gambling, sex, Internet usage, television, movies and videos.

In *Women with Attention Deficit Disorder,* Sari Solden, calls AD/HD a "hidden disorder" and beautifully describes the inner lives of women who still struggle with a healthy self-concept, though they are capable in so many ways. "Women with ADD often live in a secret world....Their inner world is a place that outsiders couldn't even fathom, where the simplest activities—getting dressed, planning the day, or running a simple errand—are extremely difficult and frustrating" (p. 50).

Without proper treatment, women with AD/HD can live a lifetime of self-loathing, under achievement, anxiety, and often even clinical depression. Women need to be more proactive and find the help they need in order to stop the cycle of misdiagnosis and "sub-optimal" treatment. The following paragraphs elaborate on some of the experiences that are routine for women with AD/HD but that are rarely directly connected with this condition.

For some women, socializing is one big can of worms with anxieties that range from simply holding their own in a conversation to knowing what to wear. Others avoid social gatherings because they tend to miss social cues, making them feel out of step and embarrassed. And the thought of entertaining at home is out of the question because of the piles of clothes, dishes, papers and assorted knickknacks.

Ultimately, many women with AD/HD suffer enormous losses in terms of developing and maintaining social connections. Intimate relationships present their own set of challenges. Many an AD/HD woman finds herself bored in an intimate relationship and sabotages it only to find herself in a similar situation with a different partner down the road. Marriages are often strained for a number of reasons. She may find it excruciating to endure certain aspects of physical intimacy due to the many hypersensitivities listed above. Even the lightest touch can cause some to react as if they are hearing fingernails scraping across a blackboard—it can literally be painful!

If a woman chooses a job that is not "AD/HD friendly", she could experience a great deal of stress. Distractions at work, procrastinating on important projects, generally feeling overwhelmed—these are all potential roadblocks to a woman advancing her career.

Parenting is just as challenging as any career but has much higher stakes: the health and well-being of those she loves most. If a woman can't organize her own life, how is she to manage her children's belongings and daily activities? Mothers who regularly "check out" while daydreaming often feel a "dis-connect" with their family. Children mistakenly interpret that as their mother not caring. When you throw the likelihood that one or more of her kids will have AD/HD into this mix, things become even more difficult.

Meal planning is another area in which women who have AD/HD typically do *not* shine, though there are definite exceptions. Some women with AD/HD are gourmet cooks; they have found a way to express their creativity in the kitchen and thrive on multi-tasking. But for most it can be an overwhelming aspect of their every day lives since it involves so many separate tasks. Think about all of the cognitive skills it requires that women with AD/HD typically struggle with:

- Making decisions: deciding on all the elements that go into a balanced meal (protein, vegetables, starches, etc.) let alone what flavors go well together!
- Memory: remembering to purchase all of the essential ingredients during the *first* trip to the grocery store.
- Hypersensitivities: feeling overwhelmed by the stimuli in the store as it floods their senses,

forcing them to race in and out as fast as they can.

• Sequencing: feeling confused when it comes to measuring, struggling to juggle the timing required to pull together two to three dishes in a short period of time, let alone courses for a larger, more formal meal.

This problem is compounded when, as is often the case, no one in the family is eager to eat what a mom has spent hours planning and preparing. Many children with AD/HD are extremely picky about what they'll eat, thus agitating an already stressed out mom with AD/HD.

With all of this to contend with, women with AD/HD need extra doses of support and knowledge. They need to ask their doctors and therapists questions or/and join support groups, including those found online such as my free online chat support for women with AD/HD: www.addconsults.com/digichat. They can read books and articles and attend conferences. Each woman must be her own best advocate for getting the help she needs. Once she's learned how AD/HD impacts her life, she can then move forward in a much healthier way.

It may be helpful to read how others made their journey from self-doubt to acceptance and how the proper treatment has helped their lives. Below are comments from women with AD/HD on how they found support through treatment, connecting with others, and education.

> Until I was diagnosed with AD/HD, I thought I was just plain stupid, even though my IQ test showed a score of 135.
>
> Tamara McKerry
> Toronto, Canada

Once I began taking medication for my AD/HD, I felt like Dorothy in *The Wizard of Oz* stepping into a world full of color for the first time.

Liz Packard
Los Angeles, CA

At the ripe old age of 52 I attended my first conference on AD/HD....everyone around me was spilling their coffee, losing their hotel key, and getting lost. I was home!

Karen Ross
Akron, OH

You know what the problems are; you've lived with them your whole life. But now you can put them into the context of your own neurology! Now you can arm yourself with innovative tools that will help you to overcome the obstacles mentioned above. It may not always be a smooth, easy road, but I hope this book carries you through some of the many bumps because with understanding comes the power to take control of your life and to live it more fully. I invite you to link arms with your "AD/HD sisters" and march forward with your chin up, knowing that you are not alone in your travels.

Chapter 3

Here, There, and Everywhere: Specifics for Organizing Your House

If you're like me, the kitchen ranks right up there with the basement when it comes to rooms I hate to spend time in! This chapter provides you with specific advice on how to organize your house. Let's start with the kitchen since, besides the bedroom, it is the place most women spend a majority of their time.

Organizing the Kitchen

Tip #1: Saving time on cleanup—use a plastic bin

> I save time going back and forth from the table to the sink with dirty dishes by keeping a plastic bin next to the table and filling it up with all the dishes, then taking them to the sink in one fell swoop. I got that idea from watching restaurant busboys. Works for me!
>
> Connie Marcus
> Cleveland, OH

Tip #2: Keeping kitchen tools tidy—consolidate!

My measuring spoons and cups used to be all over the place. Now I keep them in one big mixing bowl.

The added bonus is that it's the bowl I usually use for baking and the measuring tools are already there when I need them.

Tanya Fellows
Seattle, WA

Tip #3: Losing small jars in the fridge—use a Lazy Susan
The mornings are always insane for me and my three school-aged children. To make things easier in making their lunches every morning, I have a small Lazy Susan that I keep in the fridge, with things like jelly, mayo, and other small jars that often get lost in the shuffle. It's become my "lunch station."

Celia Anderson
St. Paul, MN

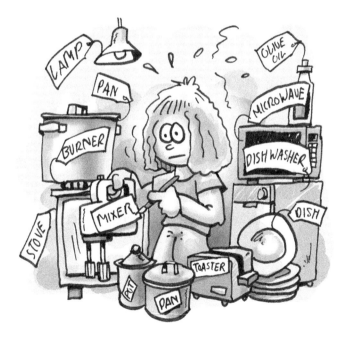

Tip #4: Finding and identifying items—label everything

This may sound crazy, but I label *everything* so that there's no mystery as to where things belong. I have labels in my pantry for things like soups, pasta, cereals, etc. I even have a white board with dry erase markers attached to my freezer, listing all the items I have inside and numbering *how many* there are of each. Then as I take food out, I update the number so that I know when it's time to buy additional food.

Sarah Randolf
Kitchener, Ontario
Canada

Tip #5: Finding room for all the food in the fridge—get creative

I never seem to have enough space in my fridge, so I try and use the space creatively. There's no law that says meats and cheese have to go in the bins. So instead, I keep our large stock of sodas and bottled waters in there. I also bought one of those small dorm-sized fridges and keep that in my kids' playroom, stocked with healthy snacks and juice.

Susan Osterman
Philadelphia, PA

Tip #6: Efficient use of space in pantry—buy expandable ledges

Buy those expandable ledges that have step ups so that you can see your items better. Things can get easily lost in the shuffle, otherwise.

Renee Constantine
Sarnia, Ontario
Canada

Tip #7: Refrigerator—new stuff in front

Always put new items in the *back* of the fridge so you use up the food in the front first. That way you don't get stuck with fermented eggs and milk because you forgot to dump out the old stuff. This rotating system has saved me lots of headaches and money!

Jen Randall
Denver, CO

Tip #8: Cupboards—Lazy Susans

Use Lazy Susans in the cupboard to stack cat food and canned foods so you can see what you have. I also use them for my spices.

Lilly Brothers
Buffalo, NY

Tip #9: Cupboards—glass vs. wood

Replace wooden doors with glass so you can see where your kitchen things are. For me, if it's out of sight, it's out of mind. I need visuals!

Lila Kadaj
Dearborn, MI

Tip #10: Placement of items—location, location, location!!!

Keep your kitchen items in logical places, e.g., pot holders near the oven, children's snacks on lower shelves, pantry items organized by frequency of use such as soup cans near the front and exotic spices in the back.

Terry Matlen

Closets, Shelves, and All the Stuff Inside!

Tip #11: Closets—managing the mess

For closets, take the doors off if possible. I do this because then I can see everything in front of me. Also, I try to keep clothes for the current season in the closet and store the rest in labeled boxes or stand-up wardrobes. It also helps to group colors together or put outfits together you know you like. Over time you may realize what you never wear. Then, you can give them away or toss them out.

Sarah Walz
Golden Valley, MN

Tip #12: Losing stuff in closets—make them visual!

ADDers are visual. If they can't see something, they won't remember they have it and will forget to use it.

- Since the top shelves of closets are *black holes*, make them smaller and save them for things you use once a year or for seasonal storage, or better yet, hang stuff from the closet ceiling and make them go away completely. Do this by putting double hanging bars in the closets and raising the top one to the highest point that you or your family member can reach—up to the ceiling if you are tall.
- Use a stacker shelf for shoes and throw the boxes away unless they are seldom-used shoes.
- Fill the ends of the closets (beyond the door openings) with wire shelving and items in plastic see-through storage boxes with lids on to use like drawers.
- Use those hanging shoe organizers for winter

19

hats and mittens and roll up the scarves; seeing them allows you to match them up easily.

- Use sliding doors rather than bi-fold doors; then at least *half* the closet is always closed to hide the mess!
- Put wire racks on the inside of the doors for small things if you have closet doors that are hinged.
- Make bookshelves, etc., just as deep as the books, no deeper. If you have 12" bookshelves for paperbacks, the front of the shelves will fill with clutter. Use adjustable shelves so that you can arrange them to fit what you need to store.

Laura Tobin
Woodstock, IL

Tip #13: Shoes—shoe bags

For shoes, over the door shoe bags or open shelving works.

Sarah Walz
Golden Valley, MN

Kids and Their Clutter

Tip #14: Keeping toys in line—use "parking spots"

When my children were smaller, we set aside "parking spots" in the playroom and family room where most of their toys landed. By the end of the day, they had to "go park their toys" in their designated spaces, which kept things basically neat.

Martha Witherspoon
Oxford, UK

Tip #15: Clutter—kids' daily room check

> My children have a room check every morning. If
> it's not straight, no videogames, no movies, no bikes,
> no swimming. That usually gets them going, and I'm
> getting better about holding the line because I don't
> get distracted by something else and forget about it,
> or give up! I also give myself a room check. If my
> shoes aren't put away, or there's a newspaper on the
> floor, a glass on the nightstand, etc., I don't get my
> privileges either! My stress/anxiety/frustration lev-
> els have decreased dramatically. I haven't had one
> depressed day this month.

Shelley Ionescu
Columbia, SC

Tip #16: Kids' clutter—make it a game

> It takes a lot of creative thinking to get kids to take
> care of their belongings, especially if they suffer from
> AD/HD, too. Here's what worked for me when mine
> were little: Play "Beat the Clock" by setting a timer
> for 10 minutes. This works even better if you have
> more than one child. The first one who gets the floor
> picked up before the timer goes off is the winner. Get
> a jar and fill it with inexpensive toys/prizes and use
> that as their reward.

Terry Matlen

Paper

Tip #17: Filing—use generic categories

> It's okay to file in large categories like "Health" and
> then place all the family members' health-related pa-
> pers under that category. It's easier to find one health-

related paper for one person among all the other health-related papers than it is to look for it all over the house—in the recycling bin, the magazine pile, the bill pile, the cut-out recipes, the latest photos, or the "I'll read these later" stuff.

Donna Parten
Sacramento, CA

Tip #18: Mail—get a shredder!
I have bought a shredder; that way each day I go through my mail as soon as I get home. I shred or throw stuff away and take care of the rest so that it doesn't build up so much although sometimes I save things to look at later.

Laura Oleson
Howard Lake, MN

Tip #19: Paper—use the trashcan
I have a trashcan right where I open the mail so I can immediately toss the junk mail out; if only the mail-man would do it for me! Then bills go straight to the bill drawer and magazines go straight to the bathroom where I will have some *time* to read them!

Sandy
Attica, IN

Tip #20: Paper work—trays
I have three trays stacked one on top of the other. If I get a bill or something that needs responding to, I put it into the top tray. Then once a week I go through the tray and clear it. Those bills or bits of paper then go to the third tray for filing. The second tray contains things that are for information or long term projects.

This helps me keep up to date as it is a visual cue for what needs doing.

Sarah M.

Tip #21: Christmas cards—be an early bird

Christmas cards—I hate doing them, so I buy them on sale and do them throughout the year. I put stamps on them and send them out in the mail December first.

Jamie Placito
Syracuse, NY

Tip #22: Magazines—file, don't pile

I love magazines but find it impossible to get rid of them for fear that I'll want to read something in the future. I read this tip somewhere and it really helps me: I tear out only the pages I want to keep (usually just a few per magazine) and stick them in a "To Read" folder. If I haven't looked at it in six months, then I toss it.

Gayle Conners
Jackson, Mississippi

Tip #23: Files—color-coding

I keep color-coded folders for these subjects: kids, home, and "to read." One folder is made of paper and is the "archive" file in my file cabinet at home; the other plastic, more durable one lives in my briefcase. Current items (for example, a flyer on skating lessons in the "kids" folder) stay in the plastic folder and are archived (in paper folder) when I've dealt with the item but need to retain the information. Using the same color (e.g., blue for kids) for the two folders makes moving items from one to the other simple and avoids cluttering my briefcase.

Karen F.

Tip #24: Kids' papers—bulletin board

I have three children which means a whole lot of school papers, reports, artwork, and more that comes home daily. I got sick of covering my fridge with everything, so I made a "Stars of the Week" bulletin board and tack up their best papers and artwork for all to admire. After a week, I save only our favorites and pitch the rest.

Amelia Wilder
Medford, OR

Tip #25: Kids' art work—portfolios

I never knew what to do with the seemingly billions of art projects and other various work my kids brought home from school until I purchased large brown art portfolios for each child and saved only the best pieces per semester year. That did the trick!

Terry Matlen

Tip #26: Storage areas—follow your instincts

I've been told by a professional organizer to *do what works for me.* To me that means I keep things I need to find in the open, in bins, or on clear plastic shelves on rolling carts. I also realize it helps to *label* these bins so I remember what's in them! *Color* helps, too. ADDers are visual, so color will catch our attention. At Target, they have colorful storage bins for children, but whatever works for us is what matters.

Sarah Walz
Golden Valley, MN

Tip #27: Keys—consistency is the "real" key

> Always keep your main set of car and door keys in the *same* outside pocket of your purse and with the rare exception, don't change purses. I put my name, home phone number, and home P.O. Box (*not* a physical address) on a small ID tag on this set as, well as on another set. Resist the temptation to temporarily put keys in a pocket, on a counter, or anywhere else. Just in case, keep a second set of car keys clipped to the inside of your purse, an ignition key hidden inside the car, and a third set of car and door keys with ID hidden on the outside of your car. If I go into the city (I live in rural area) or travel where I know I won't need office keys, this set goes onto a key organizer at home. We have a home door key hidden outside which I use for those occasions when the main set of door keys is left at home for safe keeping.
>
> Karen Robertson
> Washington

Tip #28: Keys—color-coding

> I don't know about you, but I have about a dozen keys that I drag around with me. Of course, I can never remember which key goes to which door, so I purchased a variety of plastic colored key tabs that slip right over the tops. I color code them: yellow for home, green for office, etc. You can buy these at your local hardware store.
>
> Terry Matlen

Organizing in General

Tip #29: General systems—keep it simple, sweetheart!
Keep things as simple as possible. If an organizational system takes too long to set up or maintain, it will not be used for long.

Bonnie Toering
Vancouver WA

Tip #30: General systems—think of the family!
One way that helps me to stay organized (as best I can!) and to avoid clutter is to remind myself what kind of shape my house would be in the event that I dropped dead and left this mess for my husband and kids to deal with. Sounds weird, but it does motivate me to take care of my "stuff" and also not to hoard so much.

Kristin Phelan
Warwick, RI

Tip #31: Organizing in general—plastic, coiled chains
If you have ever been to a casino, you may have noticed the long, plastic-coiled chains people use for their slot machine cards. The best thing about them is that they are free from the casinos! I saw immediately that these are handy for a *lot* of things that tend to get easily misplaced. Here are some of the uses I have found for them:

Kitchen: scissors clipped to the kitchen drawer handle.

Office: stapler clipped to my copy machine's stand. It also reaches to everywhere in my office, so no need to unclip it unless I need to remove it from that room.

Woodshop: lathe tightening/centering tool, protractor, and Dremel rotary tools. Now I can at least find *one* of the six that I have when I need one.

Truck: comb because it's a lot easier to pull something out from between the seats when you can see the chord that's attached to it. It's easier to grab my comb when in motion, too.

Shower bag: around the neck of my travel shampoo bottle because I was always leaving it behind in the truck stop shower rooms. Now it has no choice but to follow me out the door, attached to my shower bag.

Various rooms: pens attached to the computers, the phones, the bed tables, the toilets, etc. I've gotten quite used to things being tied down around me.

Front door knob: Keys. It took me about two years to get them on the *right* doorknob, but during that "training" time, my keys were a lot easier to find because I only had 20 possible doorknobs to look on instead of 100s of places I could have hidden them! The worst is when I leave them sitting in the lock outside. Well, it *is* a doorknob...but not quite the one that I had in mind. When I visit others, I also hang my keys on their doorknob so I can find them when I leave.

Crystal St. Clair
Poulsbo, WA

Tip #32: Organizing in general—eBay!

One word: eBay! We've made a nice bit of money by simply getting rid of our junk and selling it online. Our teenage son, who is very computer savvy, set up our account and handles a lot of the uploading. He earns a percentage of whatever we sell.

Tess Herrold
Santa Fe, NM

Chapter 4

Strawberry Fields:
Meals and Entertaining

I am one of many women with AD/HD whose nightmares begin upon awakening rather than during the wee hours of the night, for the first thought that comes into *my* mind when my eyes open at 6:45 AM is, *"What should I make for dinner tonight????"* The first 20 years of marriage produced daily potluck surprise—throw something in a pot and be surprised if it came out tasty enough to pass the lips of a living soul (dogs and cats excluded, of course). So in my twenty-first year of marriage, I came up with some solutions. My favorite was to stop cooking, but that one aside…

Grocery Shopping
Tip #1: Grocery store phobia—shop ahead and cook in quantity

I shop every weekend. I've had this weird phobia of grocery stores all my life and never knew why until I learned I have AD/HD. Since I started meds, I don't get so overwhelmed in there anymore, and my diet has improved a great deal since I now always have food in my cupboards. It's an effort to cook dinner for myself. It just seems so silly to cook a complete meal for just me, but sometimes I will cook up two or three pork chops and a whole batch of veggies so that the next day I can just reheat them.

Erin Gallagher
Wilkes-Barre, PA

Tip #2: Feeling overwhelmed—shop after dinner

I find that I'm not nearly as overwhelmed by grocery shopping if I go on weekday evenings after work or after dinnertime around 8:00 or 9:00 PM. Going after dinner also prevents me from "binge shopping" or buying extra items I don't really need. I shop at a smaller chain store (Dominick's in the Chicago area where I live) versus a mega-grocery chain store (Meijer, Cub Foods, Super Kmart, etc.). I also keep a small note pad in my kitchen and faithfully write down items as they are used up. As a birthday present to myself last year, I purchased an inexpensive Sony PDA (Personal Data Assistant) to keep track of important items or those on sale, in case I forget to bring my list to the store. I keep coupons in a small box organized by category with small envelopes. I often put my list and coupon box in my care the night before I plan to shop so I'm ready to go the next day.

Jolie M.

Tip #3: Tracking needed items—date everything

I'm bad at shopping, but I do keep a black marker in my kitchen and write the date on everything as I put it away. At least then I use the oldest stuff first! I got this idea from the scout quartermaster room!

Laura Tobin
Woodstock, IL

Tip # 4: Remembering what to buy—various tips

Shop at the same stores, and you'll eventually memorize where things are. Always take a list. Sit down and create a menu for three days and then shop accordingly. Buy a magnet and keep a running list of supplies on the fridge. Write items down immediately. If you forget your list, call home to get someone to read you your list. Otherwise, go to the store, park, turn the car off, sit, and try to visualize the items on the list and write it them down.

Tamara Gabrielsen
Halsey, OR

Tip #5: Running out of items—stock up

I buy toilet paper and paper towels "a package ahead;" that is I always have two or three packages in storage. When package A is gone, I open B, and make a note to buy package D. For anyone without AD/HD, this might seem obsessive. But things happen, life happens, and life is too short to be bothered by a shortage of paper goods.

Mirjam Baranihof
Lyon, France

Tip # 6: Impulsivity—prioritize before buying

When I'm grocery shopping, I tend to let my impulsivity get the better of me (especially when there are sales). As a college student, I really can't afford to buy a lot, so before I go into the checkout line, I go through *everything* in my cart to be sure it's something I absolutely need. If there's doubt in my mind, I put it back. I have tried making lists before I go and only buying things on my list, but it never seems to work. I either forget the list or forget to put important things on the list. Lists *do* help me, and I use them as much as possible but double checking the cart is a great safety measure.

Christiana D.

Cooking

Tip #7: Running out of items—grow your own herbs

Two years ago I planted lots of herbs in my garden. I really was only interested in the basil but thought it looked nice to have several others. Then last year I planted onions and garlic, primarily so that my kids could see how they grow. This has turned out to be the best thing for my cooking!!! All of my herbs except for the basil survive through the winter. The onions and garlic can be dug up when I need them (and the home-grown garlic lasts much longer once it is harvested than the store-bought garlic). Now when I flip thru a cookbook at the last minute, I don't have to pass over recipes because I forgot to buy garlic and onions, etc. It's just a quick trip outside to get what I need. Cooking is more fun, and I don't get annoyed at myself for not having been organized enough to shop for what I would need.

Nadia Carrell
Bethesda, MD

Tip #8: Forgetting food—leave microwave door open

I always leave the microwave door open so that I know there is nothing inside that I forgot to remove after the timer shut off. Yes, it *is* possible with ADHD to forget to eat. This way, there are no more dreadful surprises when I open the microwave door the next day.

Crystal St. Clair
Poulsbo, WA

Tip #9: Forgetting food on stove—timer
When cooking anything, and I mean *anything*—even boiling a couple of eggs—set a timer immediately, and take the timer with you wherever you go—*yes, even if you're going to sit on the throne, set that timer in front of you!!!!!*

Fanciulla Dell Ouest
New York, NY

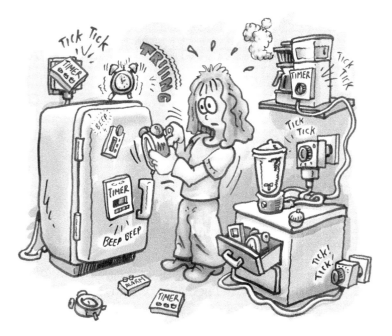

Tip #10: Not burning food—turn it off before the suggested time

To reduce the risk of incineration of both food and dwelling, turn off the stove and range before the food is fully cooked. I found that I can let some meals finish in a hot oven or on a turned off stovetop. If there's about ten minutes or so to go in the oven and I turn it off, the oven will stay hot long enough to finish baking the meal. If I have sauce or something on the stove, I put a lid on and turn off the range just before the end of the suggested cooking time. It traps the heat, finishes the cooking, and again, decreases the risk of disaster. To prevent microwave popcorn from burning, put the popcorn in for three or four minutes but listen for when the kernels stop popping as fast as they were at peak popping frequency.

T. McIntyre

Tip #11: Food preparation—bunch of anonymous tips from an old online Web site

- Wrap celery in aluminum foil and refrigerate—it will keep for weeks.
- Use lifesavers candy to hold candles in place on your next birthday cake. Kids love them!
- Poke an egg with a small sewing needle before hard-boiling, and the egg will peel with ease. And hold that needle in place with a magnet refrigerator clip.
- Stuff a miniature marshmallow in the bottom of a sugar cone to prevent ice cream drips.
- Zap garlic cloves in the microwave for 15 seconds and the skins slip right off.
- Use a meat baster to "squeeze" your pancake

batter onto the hot griddle perfectly shaped pancakes every time.

- To keep potatoes from budding, place an apple in the bag with the potatoes.
- To prevent egg shells from cracking, add a pinch of salt to the water before hard-boiling.
- Use a pastry blender to cut ground beef into small pieces after browning.
- Sweeten whipped cream with confectioners' sugar instead of granulated sugar. It will stay fluffy and hold its shape better.
- For easy "meatloaf mixing," combine the ingredients with a potato masher.
- If you don't have enough batter to fill all cupcake tins, pour one tablespoon of water into the unfilled spots. This helps preserve the life of your pans.
- Run your hands under cold water before pressing Rice Krispie treats into the pan. The marshmallow won't stick to your fingers!
- Mash and freeze ripe bananas in one-cup portions for use in later baking (or you can freeze them whole, peeled, in plastic baggies. No more wasted bananas.
- To quickly use that frozen juice concentrate, simply mash it with a potato masher. No need to wait for it to thaw. A wire whip works, also.
- To get the most juice out of fresh lemons, bring them to room temperature and roll them under your palm against the kitchen counter before squeezing.
- When a cake recipe calls for flouring the baking pan, use a bit of the dry cake mix instead. No

more white mess on the outside of the cake.
- If you accidentally over-salt a dish while it's still cooking, drop in a peeled potato. It absorbs the excess salt for an instant "fix me up."
- When making bread, substitute nondairy creamer for the dry milk. It works just as well.
- Rinse cooked ground meat with water when draining off the fat. This helps "wash away" even more fat! Use *hot* or *warm* water so the fat won't congeal.
- Slicing meat when partially frozen makes it easier to get thin slices.
- Substitute half applesauce for the vegetable oil in your baking recipes. You'll greatly reduce the fat content. (Example: 1/2 cup vegetable oil =1/4 cup applesauce + 1/4 cup oil)
- To ripen avocados and bananas, enclose them in a brown paper bag with an apple for two to three days.
- Brush beaten egg white over pie crust before baking to yield a beautiful, glossy finish.
- In recipes calling for margarine, substitute reduced-calorie margarine to help cut back on fat. Same goes with sour cream, milk, cheese, cream cheese, and cream soups.
- Place a slice of bread in hardened brown sugar to soften it back up.
- When boiling corn on the cob, add a pinch of sugar to help bring out the corn's natural sweetness.
- When starting your garden seedlings indoors, plant the seeds in eggshell halves. Simply crack the shells around the roots of your plants and transplant them outdoors. The shell is a natural

fertilizer!
- To determine whether an egg is fresh or not, immerse it in a pan of cool, salted water. If it sinks, it is fresh; if it rises to the surface, throw it away.

Meal Planning

Below are valuable tips on meal planning. For specific recipes refer to chapter 18, "Savoy Truffle: SOS Recipes."

Tip #12: Meal preparation—rice cooker

Get a rice cooker, also known as a rice/pasta/potato/ veggie cooker—it's all you'll ever need for a balanced diet. Then pick a variety of "family meal makers"— those instant food packets usually prepared on the stovetop—one for each night. Follow the directions on the back of the package but tip them all into the rice cooker together, stir, put lid on, switch to cook, walk away, and when you remember you started dinner, you'll come back to find dinner cooked and even kept warm! Buy jumbo frozen veggies to add, too, and always, always buy pre-cut chicken or meat strips—no boring chopping or peeling to do. Tuna (brain food) is great to add.

Briana
Bristol Qld. Australia

Tip #13: No time to plan—weekly menu

My husband and I work well beyond full-time hours on different shifts. We have found that meal planning and preparation is a lot less stressful if we decide a weekly menu. In the mornings, I do as much prep work as possible (cutting veggies, putting everything in the pot ready for the oven, grating cheese, etc.). He then finishes the meal and dishes are done together so that we can discuss any household issues that need to be discussed. It's always easier with two.

Cherity Kingston
Wilcox, NE

Tip #14: Can't decide on menu?—get online recipes
I subscribe to an online weekly menu. Each week I receive an email that contains six recipes and a shopping list to go with it. There are also suggestions for side dishes. What a help this is! You don't have to decide what's for dinner, what to buy at the store, or even make a list! Print off that shopping list and you're good to go. The added bonus is getting up each morning knowing what's for dinner that night.

Linda
Crystal, MI

Tip #15: Struggling with finding online recipes—how to search for online recipes
This is a tip for those with a computer and an internet connection. When I get stuck at mealtimes and can't remember what I have on hand or what ingredients a dish requires, I just do a search at Google.com. Sometimes I just type in what ingredients I have like chicken, rice, broccoli, or cheese soup, and finish with the word "RECIPE." (I was coming up with fancy menu items from famous restaurants until I stuck "RECIPE" in there.) If you are on a special diet, you can add limiters such as salt free, sugar free, fat free, low carbs, etc. Or if you primarily cook dishes associated with the cuisine of one country, you can type in

things like Italian, Southwestern, Mexican, Greek, German, etc. Or you can type in specific words such as the following: easy, crockpot, casserole, microwave, barbeque, camp stove, make ahead, vegetarian, vegan, roasting bag, foil packets, etc. If you have kids that are demanding McDonalds or other fast foods, you can try searches like Big Mac recipe, Taco Bell burrito recipe, etc. It's been very helpful to me to type in the ingredients I *have* instead of plowing through recipes only to find I don't have one or more key ingredient and becoming stressed.

Maladdees
California

Tip #16: Need something fast—SOS meals

One of my favorite SOS meals is the frozen bag that contains "everything" you need for a full meal: chicken or meat, vegetables, and if you're really lucky, a starch, like rice or noodles. VOILA! Buy two bags and dinner is on the table. You can even get away without adding a salad.

Fran Glindenberg
Baltimore, MD

Tip #17: Quickie meal—make a side dish the star

Buy large quantities of a frozen side dish you like, and make that the main dish. Instead of *one* box of mac and cheese, buy four. Add a salad or cut veggies and you're set.

Randi Walters
Atlanta, GA

Tip #18: Quickie meal—appetizers

Have an appetizer dinner: buy cocktail hotdogs in a crust (in the freezer department), Tater Tots, and if you're really feeling adventurous, slice some fruit and thread it onto skewers.

Marcie Silver
Concord, MA

Tip #19: Efficiency—freeze meals

Cook large meals and freeze leftovers in one-serving containers.

RM
Portland, OR

Tip #20: Saving time—preparation

Whenever you are cooking a meal at the stove, try to never leave a burner unused! Work at coming up with a list of ingredients that are often used in dishes you prepare. You can boil many things that can be stored in the refrigerator and be used for dishes later such as eggs (for egg or tuna salad), pasta (for pasta salad or to reheat in Microwave for hot pasta meal), potatoes (potato salad), rice (hot or cold rice dishes, rice pudding, or casseroles), bacon (cooked medium-well to be ready to zap in the microwave when needed), beans or legumes (for chili or soups), diced apples (applesauce, apple filling), etc.

Instead of just chopping enough veggies for the meal you are making, chop or dice all the celery, onions, carrots, etc. you have and use a nice compartmentalized container to store them in the fridge. These are nice to have on hand for cooking pasta salads, omelets, dinner salads, soups or casseroles. (Diced fruit is also good to have for cold/hot cereal, yogurt, smoothies, baking, and juice extracting).

I can't count the times I have settled for a sandwich because I couldn't cope with the chopping or prep cooking! This can also just be an individual project when you are not cooking. You can become your own prep-chef so that everything is ready for combining when you are ready to cook a meal!

Maladdees
California

Tip #21: Quickie meals—online recipes

There are many great online resources for cooking and meal planning. An exhaustive list is at www.ability.org.uk/food.html. For coming up with last minute ideas, you can punch in your food items at hand and up pops menu ideas: www.my-meals.com To have a weekly menu sent to you via email, check out www.recipes.com There are lots of free eNewsletters to choose from with recipes, menu ideas, and more: www.allrecipes.com/mbr/sub1.asp Here are some great sites if you're looking for quick and easy recipes:

1. www.razzledazzlerecipes.com/quickneasy/
2. www.recipeland.com/recipes/quick_easy/
3. www.allfood.com/mmeal.cfm (This one offers a game plan, a shopping list, and very specific steps.)
4. www.dianaskitchen.com/page/skillet.htm (These are meals in a skillet. Simply add a salad and you're all set.)

5. www.healthy-quick-meals.com (These are quick, healthy, easy recipes. They will also deliver seven easy dinner recipes via email when you subscribe to their free meal planner.)

Tracey Mulvaney
Paris, TX

Tip #22: Meal planning—various tips

- Carry out: if that means five days a week to maintain your sanity, go for it.
- Out of ideas? Make breakfast for dinner: scrambled eggs, waffles with fruit, etc.
- Throw ingredients in a crock-pot before you go to bed. Turn it on before leaving for work and dinner is ready when you get home. Use my "POS" (Plan or Starve) cards: For every day of the week, I have an index card with a full menu on it. By menu, I mean there is one home made course—the main dish—and ready made side dishes. If you are like me, then preparing just one part of a meal is enough to feel like an accomplished cook. My cards look like this:

MONDAY: Meatloaf, frozen peas, mashed potatoes from a box, bagged salad.

TUESDAY: Roast Chicken, canned string beans, bagged salad....and so on.

In addition to the M-F cards, (no cooking for me on Saturday or Sunday—those days are sacred) I also add a couple of Jokers (wild cards). These consist of two choices: take out or a "really" quick and easy recipe like cooked pasta with bottled spaghetti sauce, or tuna on toast, topped with cheese. You get the picture.

- Having trouble just "deciding" what to make? Get a cooking buddy and check in daily for ideas.
- Are your kids picky eaters? If you can involve them in the process, they'll be more likely to eat what's been prepared. You'd be amazed just how much a little one can help out. Also, give each child a sheet of paper and have them (with your help if they are really young) write down their favorite meals. Put them in a plastic holder and then rotate meals: one day is Johnny's choice, the next day is Amy's. Of course, *you* choose the rest of the week!
- Here's another idea. Make your own Month-of - Meals (MOM) plan, filling in each day with a simple menu *(See Appendix for a sample MOM plan)*. Of course, this is only a sample. Use your own family favorites and enlist the help of family members. You could even write each meal on a Post-It and move them around depending on your schedule, then have them handy for the next month's chart.

Terry Matlen

Entertaining

Tip #23: Pleasing guests—call ahead

If you like cooking for your friends, remember to let them know beforehand what you plan to cook so you can ask them if they might not like it. There's nothing worse than all that stressing and freaking out, only to have most of it still sitting in the serving dishes at the end of the night. Boy, do I wish my best AD/HD friend had warned me she was serving me catfish before she went to all that trouble! There will be times when you are experimenting on a new dish and didn't plan ahead to advise your guests of the menu. Feel perfectly free to announce at the table that this food is an experiment and for those who don't like it, you're prepared to feed them something else so they won't go hungry, like a sandwich. Announce this with a hearty laugh and be prepared to follow up. Check your pantry first and don't offer a peanut butter sandwich as a substitute if you have run out of peanut butter.

Donna Parten
Sacramento, CA

Tip #24: Alternative to cooking—pot lucks

If you avoid entertaining because you hate to cook or are too disorganized to pull a meal together, consider the old standby—pot lucks. If your friends hate to cook, too, make a "Take-Out Pot Luck Dinner," and instruct everyone to pick up foods from their favorite carry-out spots. Just make sure you check to see what everyone is bringing so that you don't end up with 30 buckets of Kentucky Fried Chicken.

I actually *had* to have a pot luck once. I had invited 12 people over for a holiday dinner but just hours before their arrival found that I had forgotten all of the carry-out food I'd bought and had left it in my hot car for hours. It was too spoiled to use, so I called up all my friends and told them to bring over their left-overs. We ended up having a smorgasbord holiday dinner. Clever, I guess but totally unintended!

Terry Matlen

Chapter 5

Fixing a Hole:
How to Delegate, Eliminate,
and Simplify Household Chores

Keeping on top of the laundry pile can be exasperating. If the laundry room is in the basement, it's easy to forget about laundry entirely: out of sight, out of mind! Although it *seems* like a simple enough task, think of the complexity of all the steps involved: sorting, washing, drying, folding, and putting things away. Again, memory becomes an issue—remembering to *do* the laundry, taking it *out* of the washer before it begins to smell of basement rot, and remembering the boring job of putting things away. These tips should help you along with this endless chore.

Laundry

Tip #1: Lost socks—sock pins

Use brass safety pins (if you use the silver ones they rust) to attach everyone's matching socks prior to the wash and then throw them into the dryer, as well. I leave some on each of the kids' dressers and some in the bathroom near the hamper. When the wash is completed, they are all sorted. The kids actually like doing this and even unpin them when its time to wear them.

Lisa M. Pomerantz
Danvers, MA

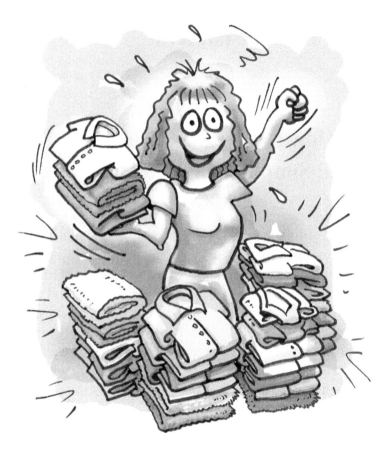

Tip #2: Putting laundry away—various tips

The worst part of laundry for me is putting it away, so as soon as I empty the dryer, I have a closet rod hanging over the washer and dryer with hangers on it, so I hang up stuff immediately. I have a sock basket sitting on top of the dryer to toss socks in, and I fold everything and place it all on top of the washer. In order to put the laundry from the washer to the dryer, I have to unload the washer so that forces me to put the dried clothes in the dryer away first. The closet rod is hung low enough that I have to put that stuff away, too, or I won't have room to put stuff. Then when the sock basket is full, I sort those and put them away.

Sandy
Attica, IN

Tip #3: Lost uniform socks—separate

Soccer socks get washed in a separate load with the travel soccer uniform so they don't get lost in the wash. Similar for baseball—either buy a bunch of the baseball socks or keep them separate with the baseball uniform shirts for washing.

Cathlin Darling-Owen
Vermont

Tip #4: Getting it all done—hang right out of the dryer

I don't have a washer/dryer and have to go to a laundromat to do laundry. It is a huge effort, and I often put it off until I had six loads to do. Then I'd get home and be so sick of looking at laundry that I would never put the clean clothes away. I would live out of the laundry basket, put the dirty clothes on the floor, and usually end up with everything in wrinkles so I would be constantly ironing something to wear. My solution is to *make* myself go to the laundromat every weekend. Also, I take hangers to the laundromat and put my work clothes on hangers as soon as they come out of the dryer. Then when I get home, I hang them up immediately in my closet. Sometimes I still slack on putting away the socks and undies, etc., but it's a system that seems to be working for me.

Erin Gallagher
Wilkes-Barre, PA

Tip #5: Laundromat—various tips

For laundry, I have two dirty clothes baskets: one for light colors, warm water wash, and one for dark colors and cold water wash. If you have to use a laundromat, put your soap, bleaches, and dryer sheets in a container together so that you don't forget any of them. It also makes it easier to carry them to the car. I also have a cup to put my laundromat change in.

Tamara Gabrielsen
Halsey, OR

Tip #6: Save time—Shout Color Catcher (dye catcher for the washer)

Another thing that helps me with laundry is a product called the Shout Color Catchers. They are little dye-catching sheets that prevent clothes from turning colors if you've accidentally tossed in clothes that "bleed." This way I can toss whites, colors, etc. into the wash with one of those and they all come out the correct color!! This also saves time sorting. Here's the URL:: www.shoutitout.com/family_catcher.html

Sandy
Attica, IN

Tip #7: Matching socks—buy "unibrand" socks

Only buy the same kind of socks. Buy 12 packs if

necessary – be boring and stick with all white same brand and all black same brand. I even bought my seven-year-old and nine-year-old the same socks so we'd have less trouble. This way matching socks becomes much, much easier.

Cathlin Darling-Owen
Dummerston, VT

Cleaning and Decluttering

Tip #8: Time for chores—Fly Lady and timer

One of the biggest things that has helped me is the website www.flylady.net. She speaks a lot of breaking things down into little jobs, e.g., "Set the timer for 15 minutes and do the task at hand." Her motto is that anyone can do anything for 15 minutes. For 15 minutes, I'll work at cleaning the kitchen. When the timer goes off, I'll set it for 15 minutes and straighten up the living room. Then for 15 minutes, I'll fold laundry. Then for 15 minutes I take a break and play with the kids or simply, just take a break. When I spend just 15 minutes in one zone, I see some accomplishment which encourages me to do more, or at least keep that clean. And when I get behind, I try not to beat myself up and spend all night catching up. I just spend 15 minutes doing one little job and see what I can accomplish. It has really been a lifesaver for me.

LeAnn
Albany, OR

Tip #9: Save time—basket method

We all have those occasions when company is coming and our house is a wreck. Don't despair—use the laundry basket method. Simply use a couple of large laundry baskets and go around the house putting everything that needs to find a home into the basket. Then stuff the baskets into a closet and shut the door. Now you are ready to dust, sweep, and make the place look presentable in just a few minutes. Just make sure to put the guests coats on a bed and not in the aforementioned closet, and no one will be the wiser!

Julie
Clarksville, MD

Tip #10: Too much stuff—purging
The simplest but most effective thing I have done is to reduce the amount of stuff there is to organize. Too much stuff creates noise in my head!! To this end, I have started paring down my possessions: unread books have gone to charity shops, clothes not worn for six months are out, knick-knacks are ditched, even the kids toys are down to a few well-loved favourites—simplicity is the key for me.

Lilith
Bristol, UK

Tip #11: Unwanted items—bag them!
I keep a large plastic garbage bag on the inside door-knob of my upstairs linen closet. Whenever I come across clothes that my kids have outgrown, or household items that can be given to charity, I just dump them into the bag. I have a charity truck come by on a regular basis, which motivates me to keep tossing things into that bag.

Terry Matlen

Tip #12: Staying focused—one chore at a time

I have to do one chore at a time and follow through. Usually I pick up the house first, then I vacuum, dust, sweep, and mop, but I really have to make sure I stay focused or else I will get distracted and start something in every room and never finish any of them.

Juanita K Wilkins
Houston, TX

Tip #13: Feeling overwhelmed—get a housekeeper

A cleaning person once a week for three hours has made a huge difference for me. One, it forces me to organize some things before s/he comes. Two, it maintains a basic level of cleanliness that would cost me huge amounts of concentration and energy. Money is very tight, and I've had to cut a lot of other expenditures in order to afford this, but the cleaning person is the last thing I would give up. The only challenge has been to keep the cleaning person from "straightening things up" that really, truly need to be left in the piles I'm working on.

Mirjam Baranihof
Lyon, France

Tip #14: Staying focused—teamwork and a clutter cart

Honestly, the only way my house gets clean is if I've invited people over. When we do clean, it really helps me stay focused and get a lot done if my husband and I work as a team. We work on the same room together, so it's also a social time. I get less distracted, and he not only motivates me but encourages me as we get things uncluttered and cleaned!

Try using a big plastic "tote" for items that don't belong in each room, i.e., clutter. Set a kitchen timer for 15 minutes and do a "sweep" of the house by taking the tote from room to room and filling it with misplaced items. You can do this in two steps. First, fill up the tote. Then, take a break for 20 minutes. Then, empty it by taking it from room to room, putting things back where they belong. It keeps my house less cluttered! The problem is that I don't have a designated home for everything! Then what?

Sarah Walz
Golden Valley, MN

Dishes

Tip #15: Silverware—group together

When loading the silverware into the dishwasher, I group knives, large and small forks, and spoons together. Then when I unload the silverware, it's mostly sorted. Tip: take a little care so that items don't *spoon* or nestle together too closely, as that might prevent cleaning.

Donna R.N.
Encinitas, CA

Tip #16: Baby bottles—rice bath

Put some lukewarm water in spent baby bottles and throw in some rice. Put the top back on and shake. All the nasty milk will rinse right away. For really tough jobs, it may take two tries, but the enzymes in the rice will break down the spoiled milk!!!

Amanda E. Cook

Tip #17: Staying focused—go in a circle

I find that when cleaning the kitchen, my eyes go from one area to another, and my body follows. To stay on task, eye one corner of the kitchen, clean that, then go clockwise (or counter- clockwise), de-cluttering and cleaning till you've gone full cycle.

Terry Matlen

Tip #18: Cleaning—anonymous tips from an old online Web site

- Spray your Tupperware with nonstick cooking spray before pouring in tomato-based sauces. No more stains!
- Always spray your barbecue grill with nonstick cooking spray before grilling to avoid sticking.
- To easily remove honey from a measuring spoon, first coat the spoon with non-stick cooking spray.
- To easily remove burnt on food from your skillet, simply add a drop or two of dish soap and enough water to cover bottom of the pan and bring to a boil on the top of the stove. The skillet will be much easier to clean now.
- Transfer your jelly to a small plastic squeeze bottle. No more messy sticky jars or knives. This also works well for homemade salad dressing.
- To aid in washing dishes, add a tablespoon of baking soda to your soapy water. It softens hands while cutting through grease.
- Next time you need a quick ice pack, grab a bag of frozen vegetables out of your freezer. No more watery leaks from a plastic baggie!

For a comprehensive list of tips on how to keep a kitchen clean, see the appendices.

Errands

Tip #19: Simplifying errands—group them by location
> When I have a lot of running around to do, I make a list of all the places I need to go, then group them by geographical location. I save time and gas that way.
>
> LaToya Green
Pittsburgh, PA

Tip #20: Staying focused—cooler for the unexpected delays
> Keep a cooler in your trunk for those days you get side-tracked after grocery shopping and need to keep your perishables fresh.
>
> Amanda Reynolds
Nashville, TN

Tip #21: Motivation—early bird approach
> I hate running errands so I try and get them done first thing in the morning after dropping the kids off to school. That way I'm done with it and don't have to stop what I'm doing later to run out and about.
>
> Candice Strauss
Winchester, UK

Tip #22: Staying focused—Post-its
> How many times have you gotten side-tracked running here and there and forgotten the real reason for leaving the house? I take Post-its with my destinations and lists of what I need and slip them in the crack of the steering wheel.
>
> Terry Matlen

Miscellaneous Chores

Tip #23: Feeling overwhelmed—keep basic rooms clean

Try to keep just the kitchen, living room, dining room, and one bathroom clean in order to allow friends to visit and not feel overwhelmed with the mess.

Cathlin Darling-Owen
Vermont

Tip #24: Managing distractions—master list

When cleaning, I tend to start on one thing in one room and get distracted and then go to another room and forget what I am doing. So I made a master cleaning list in which I list each room and what chores need to be done in that room. Then, I separate it, matching chores to a day of the week. After I am done with a chore, I mark off what I've done and go to the next item. I just print one list off my computer each week so my house is clean all the time; and I no longer have major cleaning once a week or four hour cleaning days.

GW

Tip #25: Sequencing and prioritizing chores—cube system

Sometimes I wear one *hat* in the house, and sometimes I wear another. When I wear the managerial hat, I set things up to be done. For example, I take the laundry to the washer/dryer, take a stack of papers to be filed to the office, or clear off the table after supper. The *trick* is to make certain that each day I take off that *managerial* hat and put on my *employee* hat. Once I am out of the conceptual/managerial way of thinking, I then tackle the laundry, the dishes, the filing, etc., coping with the details with a fresh frame of mind!

Rose Heath
Birmingham, AL

Tip #26: Keeping track—check list

I have made a list of chores for each room and had it laminated so that I can check off what I have done and then finish what I haven't gotten done the next day. This also helps me to focus on one job at a time, or else I run around doing fifty things at a time and not getting anything accomplished.

Cherity Kingston
Wilcox, NE

Tip #27: Scheduling—daily chores

Assign certain household chores to the same day each week.

Tamara Gabrielsen
Halsey, OR

Tip #28: Staying focused—timer

I use a cooking timer to stay focused on a chore. For example, I set it for 30 minutes. If the chore isn't quite done, then I can set it for another 15 minutes. I do not leave that room or that chore until the timer has gone off. This has been an absolutely marvelous tool for me. I no longer jump from room to room not accomplishing anything. It is amazing how much you can get done on one chore in 30 minutes time.

Karen Roberts
Yuma, AZ

Tip #29: Plants—water them first thing

> To help the plants survive, make it a habit to water the plants first thing in the morning every day, whether it's needed or not. It's good for you, too, to have at least one daily habit, and it helps to calm you down while you think of what day it is and what you need to do.

Siesta
Sweden

Tip #30: Plants—automatic watering device

> Use a Plant Waterer (see www.myADDstore.com) that dispenses water automatically so that you don't have to worry about plants drying out and dying.

Terry Matlen

Tip #31: Return items—basket by door

Place an errand basket by the door for library books, videos, film to be processed, etc.

Connie Engel
Bayfield, Ontario
Canada

Chapter 6

She's a Woman: Personal Tips on Clothes Shopping, Health, Hypersensitivities, and Leisure Time

Women love to go clothes shopping. Or do they? Women with AD/HD can find it a particularly daunting task—there are so many decisions to make! But filling the closet is just the first step. How often has a woman with AD/HD looked in her closet and felt like she has nothing to wear? Could it be partly that she hasn't had the time or energy in years to face decluttering her closet so that she can put her hands on *what* she needs *when* she needs it? And then there is the whole nightmare of combining separates to make an outfit. Don't you wish all clothing came with a tag that read "No Assembly Required?"

Shopping is just one aspect of self-care that women with AD/HD struggle with. Finding time for rest, relaxation, and a healthy lifestyle falls to the bottom of the list for most women but add to that women with AD/HD who struggle with *scheduling* these things, and it is easy to see why this area presents an exceptional challenge. Couple that with the many hypersensitivities women with AD/HD report, and it's no surprise that they often collapse at the end of the day. Read on to find out how other women have found strategies for simplifying while embracing their lives.

Clothes: Shopping and Dressing

Tip #1: Keeping it simple—group by color

It's easier (and less expensive) to put outfits together if you buy within the same color groups. For example, in the winter, buy all black basics. Use colors that contrast for accessories or clothing to match, e.g., black pants with a red, blue, or pink sweater. This way you don't have drawers and closets full of things that don't match! Keep a brief list in your wallet of items you need to purchase.

Tamara Gabrielsen
Halsey, OR

Tip #2: Shopping for the family—keep a list of sizes

I keep a list of sizes the family is currently wearing in my wallet so if I happen to run into a sale, I don't have wonder what size to buy.

Cherity Kingston
Wilcox, NE

Tip #3: Finding your "look"—what to wear

Make an appointment with a professional and get a list of what you look good in and what you don't. Keep it in your wallet. Alternatively, watch reality shows like "What Not to Wear" and "Style Court" and study the people who have bodies and coloring like yours.

Donna Parten
Sacramento, CA

Tip #4: Simplicity—the classic suit

All my creativity and resistance to being boring aside, I surrendered to suits. My workhorse suits have both a skirt and trousers. For some occasions or meetings, one is more appropriate than the other. Furthermore, "bottoms" show wear more quickly than jackets do, so this prolongs the life of the suit. When one piece needs dry-cleaning, oops, all the pieces go. Though not frequent, this is expensive but essential since it keeps all the pieces the same shade. In clothes/wardrobe building, focus on quality and cornerstone pieces; that is the key for me.

I don't have many clothes, but what I do have, works very hard. I've "sacrificed" a lot of fun items that only matched one other piece, and I dress very simply now. For that, I've gained a lot of peace of mind and assurance that what I am wearing is appropriate.

Mirjam Baranihof
Lyon, France

Tip #5: Coordinating outfits—index cards

Figuring out what goes together has always been a nightmare for me. Now I keep an extra large index card in my closet in full view and write down what tops go with what bottoms, where I wear them, and what accessories go with them. Since I present at lots of conferences and most have special events associated with them, my list may look something like this:

- Afternoon presentation: black suit, white cotton top, black flats, silver pendant
- Black tie dinner affair (winter): black chiffon

one piece from Saks, silk Oriental jacket, black heels, pearls

Terry Matlen

Tip #6: Staying focused—decide ahead of time
Decide exactly what you need before going (e.g., calf-length washable casual black skirt). Select the stores that are most likely to carry the item and only go into those stores. Do not browse through unrelated departments. Do not enter other stores. If necessary, take someone with you who will keep you focused or shop just prior to an appointment you must keep. If you do not need a specific item, do not enter a store at all.

Donna Parten
Sacramento, CA

Tip #7: Mix and match shopping—Chico's
I have so many clothes and never have anything to wear. I always have a mess on my hands. Then I found Chicos. Chicos is a great store that has everything that mixes and matches and is easy care. I now can buy a whole outfit (clothing, jewelry, etc.) in one place. The clothes always look great, and it has made my life so easy in the morning when I am getting ready. I only buy outfits now, never pieces that I have nothing to go with. This has been a real plus in my life since I work outside the home and have three children.

Jeannine L.

Tip #8: Creating outfits—personals shoppers
Most upscale department stores have personal shop-

pers who will put together looks for you, like a stylist. It is usually free or pretty cheap. Good for events and professional clothes, but they will do everyday clothes as well.

Andrea C.
Houston, TX

Health

Tip #9: Remembering to take meds—beeping pillboxes

You can purchase pill boxes that beep to remind you to take your meds. (An excellent one can be found at www.myADDstore.com. Just search using the word "Pill Box Timer.")

Terry Matlen

Tip #10: Getting behind in the morning—try timing yourself

Getting from bed to seatbelt every morning can take forever...or even more frightening, only a few minutes. Anxiety reigns in either predicament. Do you ever find yourself taking forever to shower, shampoo, and brush your teeth as anxiety keeping you in a racing state of hyperventilation, constantly checking the atomic clock that glares impassionately over your bathroom sink? In your mind you begin frantically retracing your tasks of the shower routine: Did I remember to put shampoo in my hair, or did I forget and just stick my head under the shower head? Did I scrub my feet, between my toes, and use the Loofah on my heals (to hell with the Loofah), and rinse out the shampoo, redoing each step without the distraction of emptyheadiness? Solution? Assign a spot on your shower in descending order for each step of your shower, and like setting a trip odometer, clock yourself. How long does each step take? Pay attention!

Mecklin
Hattiesburg, MS

Tip from Terry
Regarding exercise, Dr. John Ratey is fond of describing it as "Miracle-Gro for the brain."

Tip #11: Remembering to exercise—using a PDA

Being ADD, is it any wonder that I forget to exercise? Duh. I mark a reminder in my daily planner for the same time every day. If you use a PDA, you could program it to beep when it's time to put on your running shoes.

Janie Wilkie
Lafayette, LA

Tip #12: Motivation to exercise—buddy system

I am online a lot and have made many online buddies. We help each other get motivated for things like cleaning, chores, and exercise. One thing that has helped me a *lot* is to check in on the computer with my buds and set a time a few days a week that we exercise. When we're done, we log in again and share our exercise victories. Works for me!

Elizabeth Brown
Wilmington, DE

Tip #13: Beating exercise boredom—alternate activities

I hate exercising. It takes me away from other things I'd rather be doing, *but*...I *do* know that when I'm done, I feel incredibly renewed and my mind is clearer.

I also sleep way better at night. But the boredom of exercising is tough; I have a hard time staying motivated. So one way around that is to do something different. One day I may swim, then I ride my bike another day. If the weather is bad, I'll pop in an exercise video (make sure you have a variety!) and work out in front of the TV. I end up doing that a lot in the winter, so I try and do it early in the morning; that frees me from obsessing about it for the rest of the day.

Heidi Bates
Carmel, IN

Tip #14: Relaxation—deep breathing

This may sound stupid, but my tip is to breath. When I'm over stimulated and overwhelmed, I find a quiet spot, sit down, close my eyes, and take a really slow deep breath. (Don't do it fast; you'll get dizzy.) I keep this up until I feel centered again. This really helps me out when I'm being pulled in ten directions at once by kids and obligations. If you can't find a quiet spot, go into the bathroom!

Pamela Jean Bendel
Crystal Lake, IL

Hypersensitivities

Tip #15: Hypersensitivity to noise—use white noise

Noises bother me. My son is AD/HD, too, and he whistles, hums, sings, taps, or thumps constantly. It drives me nuts! Soft music or headphones at home and work help me concentrate and ignore outside noise. But it has to be something without words or I start singing or humming along, too! A *white noise* machine helps, or the soft sounds of the filter and air pump we have in our three fish tanks work like a white noise machine, and the fish are calming. Nothing stops that ear-piercing whistle, though, except duct tape! {*Shudder*}

Laura Tobin
Woodstock, IL

Tip #16: Hypersensitivity to noise—"No noise" rule
I hate the noise of TVs, radios, and CDs when I'm trying to eat. With a large and loud ADD family, I have a "no noise" rule at mealtime. We also take phones off the hook and let the answering machine voice mail pick up calls.

Ann Becker
Jackson, WY

Tip #17: Hypersensitivities—let others know
When I have PMS, it seems that all of my ADD symptoms worsen. I am more sensitive emotionally and just way more intolerant of noise, commotion, and even touch. I alert my family that they need to stay clear during these days. I also sometimes have to adjust my meds.

Carla Lopez
Queens, NY

Tip #18: Hypersensitivity to noise—earplugs
I wear those little spongy earplugs around the house. I have three children under the age of seven (and am guessing that at least two have ADD) so the noise level really gets to me. Since they don't block out the noise

completely, I'm still able to hear my kids. They're just a little...muffled.

Kay Miller
Spokane, WA

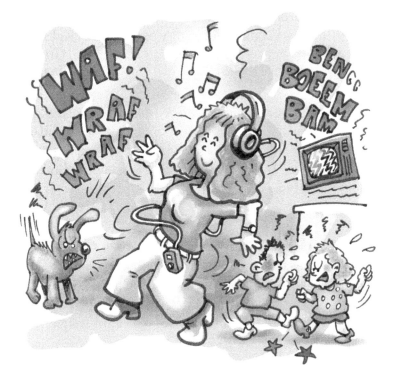

Tip #19: Hypersensitivity to fabric—accept it and accommodate

All these years, I thought I was *nuts* because I have to wear cotton clothes. I'll even wear a cotton t-shirt under my sweaters, blouses, etc. Wool makes me itch and distracts me to no end. I hate slacks with zippers or snaps and search for elastic waists. I don't care where I go; I refuse to wear panty hose. I'd rather be

69

fired from a job than have to deal with those. I also can't tolerate heels. I keep a pair of tennis shoes at work; luckily I am at a desk most of the day, so no one cares what my feet look like. Oh, I and I have to wear socks with no toe seams and I cut out every tag that is on my clothes. Now that I've learned that these traits are common in ADD women, I don't feel so bad!

Meghan Grinhardt
Sioux Falls, SD

Tip #20: Hypersensitivity to fabric—one stop shopping
You can find tagless t-shirts, seamless socks, and other "gentle" clothes for the hypersensitive at www.myADDstore.com and search under "Clothes for the Hypersensitive."

Terry Matlen

Tip #21: Hypersensitivity to fabric—one stop shopping
I hate feeling confined in clothes, especially winter coats. Is there a law that says you have to wear a coat in winter? I buy down vests with zippered pockets and wear layers of soft cotton or light-weight fleece underneath. Works for me!

Dierdre Gilpatrick
Dublin, Ireland

Tip #22: Hypersensitivity to noise—digitize!
My hearing is so sensitive, I can hear clocks and watches ticking. I hate that! So they all have to be digital, or I go out of my mind.

Jean Crane
Southfield, MI

Tip #23: Hypersensitivity to touch—communicate what you need

Certain touch really bothers me, so I have to tell my partners what feels good and what doesn't. Usually, it's just the opposite of what they expect. For instance, light touch on my skin HURTS! To get me "in the mood", there's nothing better than a nice deep head or foot massage.

Melissa McKenzie
Cambridge, MA

Tip #24: Hypersensitivity to touch—the old handshake trick

Wow, I've been reading about ADD and am relieved to know that I'm not the only one who hates being touched or hugged without warning. I swear I could punch someone out for that. I also hate it when I'm touched by strangers, so I get around this by extending my hand quickly for a handshake so that I can avoid the dreaded hug. And I thought I was nuts!?

Cammie Arrington
Orlando, FL

Tip #25: Hypersensitivities—great article

Mary Jane Johnson, ADD coach and ADDA board member, wrote a wonderful article on the connection between ADD and hypersensitivities. You can read it here: www.addconsults.com/articles/full.php3?id=1439

Terry Matlen

Tip #26: Hypersensitivities—know you're not alone

I'm not sure I have the solutions to these things but since they annoy me to no end, I thought I'd share them so that your readers wouldn't think they were crazy:

- I can't tolerate sticky floors. If there's one spill from soda or other sticky substance, I mop the floor a dozen times to get it off.
- I can't wear jewelry, especially around my neck. Though scarves aren't much better, at least they are softer and lighter. I wear those when I have to dress up.
- I have to order drinks with no ice. I hate things that are either too cold or too hot.
- Am I the only one who hates to get her face wet in the shower? I have to put a washcloth over my face!
- I have to keep my fingernails trimmed short, otherwise I can't seem to handle paper or even use the computer.
- Florescent lights make me feel sick. I avoid them as best I can.
- Perfume makes me gag.
- Believe it or not, the sound of people eating turns my stomach. Sometimes I hum in between bites or leave the room if I can get away with it.
- I hate greasy hand and face creams so I look for water-based ones.
- There's nothing worse than touching a greasy doorknob. Ugh!!
- I hate flip flops that have those things in between your toes.
- I also hate walking barefoot.

Shawna Hawthorne
Ashland, KY

Tip #27: Hypersensitivity to noise—cell phones

I absolutely cannot hear what people are saying on the other end of the phone if I'm in a room with people talking, even if they are whispering. I've switched all of my phones to cordless so that I can leave a noisy room to talk in peace.

Mindy Schwartz
Los Angeles, CA

Sleep

Tip #28: Falling asleep—relax from the toes up

This has worked for me since I was a child, when my mother taught me this method:

Start with your toes, telling them to relax, relax, relax. Then work yourself up to every body part, feeling your muscles untighten while also focusing on your breathing. Often, by the time you get to your head, you're already in la-la land.

Theresa LaFont
Fort Worth, TX

Tip #29: Falling asleep—meds before bed

I simply cannot shut my brain down. It goes like a train off a track 24/7. Much to my surprise, my doctor suggested taking another but smaller dose of my daily stimulant medication a few hours before bedtime. This has been a huge help in slowing down my brain so I can fall asleep.

Donna Landner
Las Vegas, NV

> **Note from Terry**
> Always discuss medication issues with your
> physician.

Tip #30: Falling asleep—fan
> This one works like a dream (pardon the pun). Buy a
> small floor or table fan and use it even in the winter. I
> sleep like a baby now.
>
> Mai Ito
> Tokyo, Japan

Tip #31: Getting to sleep—write out your worries
> It's easy enough to say, "I'm going to bed;" it's harder
> to actually get some sleep. Being a student requires
> that I have as much rest as possible, especially before
> an exam. In order to keep my mind from burdening
> me too much with static, I sit at my laptop for an hour
> or so before I turn in. I free write everything that's
> going through my mind, ignoring grammar and sen-
> tence structure. By the time I'm done, I've recorded
> most of the rants and annoyances of my day. This al-
> lows me to get to sleep sooner than normal because
> my subconscious knows that the information is al-
> ready recorded somewhere so there's no need to store
> it in the great windstorm of my mind.
>
> Jennifer B.

Miscellaneous
Tip #32: Keeping track of personal hygiene items—stock up
> I have saved myself a lot of time and energy by ac-
> cepting that I need to have more than one of every-
> thing. e.g., eye drops, scissors, chewing gum, what-
> ever. I just sigh and put an extra one where I might

want it because otherwise I'll be running all over the house looking for it. Every coat and jacket has a hat, gloves, lip balm, and pack of gum in the pockets. I buy three bottles of eye drops for my contact lenses. One goes on the living room table where I read the paper, one lives next to my bed, and the other is on the dresser ready to go into the pocket of whatever I'm wearing the next day. There's a comb in the car, in my pocketbook, in my computer backpack, and in my gym bag. And when I buy things like antacids, anti-inflammatories, and waterless hand cleaner, I buy the biggest size and split it up into three or four smaller containers and put them where I'm most likely to use them such as the car, upstairs, downstairs, or my backpack.

Rachel R. Peine
Levittown, PA

Travel

Tip #33: Tracking items—jackets

I used to lose my tickets and passport every time I used them and had to hunt through various pockets of bags. Even if I only had one shoulder bag and one carry-on bag, and each of them only had one "special place" for key items, it was too confusing for me. Now for travel, I always wear a jacket or a coat that has an inside pocket that holds my passport and tickets. No matter what, I always put my tickets and my passport back in this pocket. Most men's jackets have inside-chest pockets, but I haven't yet found them in women's wear. A tailor can add a patch pocket to a lining for about ¤12-20. A fancier pocket costs more.

Mirjam Baranihof
Lyon, France

Tip #34: Remembering it all—head to toe check list

When I have to pack my traveling bag kit, I think from my head down to the toes:

- Head needs brush, comb, shampoo, conditioner
- Eyes need spectacles, eye makeup
- Lips need lipstick, Chapstick
- Ears need earrings
- Body needs clothes
- Hands need pen, organizer, diary
- Feet need shoes, etc.

Anonymous

Leisure Time

Tip #35: Vacations

Vacations both from school/college or work can turn out to be an awful time for a woman with ADHD…but especially when she doesn't have kids or a family to take care of. It's just too much spare time (considering that many of us are convicted workaholics—a consequence of the constant stimulation seeking), and it can easily trigger depression. Here's my survival tip: find yourself a hobby, something you really enjoy doing, like writing, painting, or even gardening, or enroll in a language, music, an art course. What I'm saying is, keep yourself busy with some activity you really enjoy instead of feeding negative thoughts like "Oh, what can I do to kill some time right now? I feel so lost." The negative thoughts may become a very tricky way that your subconscious mind finds to kill the spare time. And you really don't want this to happen, do you?

Renata Moutinho
Rio de Janeiro/RJ/Brazil

Tip #36: Sitting still—take up a hand craft

I find that lots of women have difficulty sitting still, spending time with their spouses watching TV, etc. Many *can* if they keep their hands busy, so they might consider taking up knitting, crocheting, or some other activity that will keep their hands busy but won't require their full focus.

Terry Matlen

Setting Goals and Completing Projects

Tip #37: Reaching goals/making decisions—using pro/con lists

Making lists such as "plus/minus" or "pros/cons" has helped me make many decisions and changes in my life. On a full-size legal pad, using only the top side of each sheet, I freehand draw a line down the middle and label the top: "plus/minus" or "pro/con." There is no time limit. This project is ongoing until the decision I need to make becomes obvious to me. If I find an item on the list that I should give greater weight to in my decision-making, I give it an asterisk or underline it. If something I've written has no relevance, I cross it out. I never rewrite the list; I simply continue it onto another page. Writing this kind of list helps me focus on what I am *racketing* (tossing back and forth like a tennis ball) that is keeping me from making my decision. The list forces me to go into my gut and, at the same time, look at my reasoning more objectively. If there are several options, I give each option a pro/con or plus/minus page of its own. Once you've identified your goals, you might start another list of people and resources who will help you achieve your goals—be sure to be specific.

Here's an example of how list making helped me. I used to fantasize about having a "mother's helper" when I finally realized that help was available in my own house, but it was up to me to make it happen. I wrote up one list of what I needed someone else to do between the hours of 5:00 to 8:30 PM. Then I wrote a second list of all the things I did for my kids. The next day I read both lists aloud to my boys and told them I would agree to continue to do all the things I already did *if* they would become responsible for the chores on my want list. Not having much choice, they agreed. Next we figured out who could/would do what. This worked so well that the next year I taught them all how to sew on buttons, hem their pants, and iron a little. I never told them I hated these tasks. I was happy to get the help I needed.

Barb Golds
W. Bloomfield, MI

Tip #38: Accomplishing projects—use a master list
I keep lists of things I need to accomplish so that I don't have a million unfinished projects laying around. I don't begin new projects until I finish the ones on my list. I would have a Post-it hanging from my nose if it would stick!

Tamara Gabrielsen
Halsey, OR

Tip #39: Accomplishing tasks—visualizing
Every night before I fall asleep, I go over in my head what I'm going to make for dinner the next day or

will pick a chore from a mental list of my to-do's, like organizing a closet. The next day, if I finish my task, I treat myself to something special.

Sarah Rosen
Miami, FL

Chapter 7

I Should Have Known Better: School and Studying

One of the most frustrating aspects of being an intelligent, capable woman with AD/HD is how dumb it can make you feel, particularly in an academic environment. You know you have brilliant ideas for your term paper, but you lost your lecture notes—again! You can only use your dog's voracious appetite as an excuse so many times before the worst thing of all happens—you begin to doubt your own capabilities. We have lost the precious contributions of many gifted women with AD/HD because they either underachieved or dropped out of school before getting help. These tips are not only helpful for adult women in school or those returning to school but for our AD/HD children as well.

Study Strategies
Tip #1: Time for homework—give yourself breathers
> In college, schedule your classes an hour apart so you can do your homework in between classes at school.
>
> RM
> Portland, OR

Tip #2: Concentrating—light things up!

One thing I do is have tons of little lamps or lights in a room. I absolutely cannot concentrate with an overhead light! Our living room is 20' x 10', and I have (not counting Christmas lights) 11 or more lights in that area alone: furniture lamps, floor lamps, ceiling fan lamps, accent lighting over pictures, accent lighting on bookshelves, etc.

Rose Heath
Birmingham, AL

Tip #3: Retention—repetition

You might try reading things more than once to get it. I read a book about pregnancy, birth, and the care of babies three times through before I had my twins. I was an expert by the time they were born.

Tamara Gabrielsen
Halsey, OR

Tip #4: Note-taking—color and variety

When studying, put your class notes on one side of the page in one color and put your book notes on the other side of the page in another color. Learn different methods of studying such as visual, written, and audio.

Jamie
Syracuse, NY

Tip #5: Using time efficiently—tapes and cards

Tape a lecture and listen to it while driving. Also, you can keep 3"x 5" study cards with you at all times so that you can study while waiting in line.

RM
Portland, OR

Tip #6: Remembering and focusing—track papers with email

> I email my papers to my school email account as a backup in case I forget to bring the papers to school; then I can print them off there in proper format, etc. I email myself reminders, also.
>
> Most of all, I tend to concentrate on whatever area in life I need most at the time. It seems that I can keep things together very well either at school or at home but not both at once. The academic life is good for me because I concentrate on school and teaching during the semester and then use the breaks to catch up.
>
> Darla Wells
> Lafayette, LA

Academic Difficulties

> **Tip from Terry**
> In *ADD and the College Student*, edited by Patricia Quinn, M.D, contributors Anne McCormick, M.Ed. and Faith Leonard, Ph.D. point out the following:
>
> Organization of time and place is a major problem for many students at the college level and beyond. Frequently, it is the very freedom from structured time craved by the student that becomes a nemesis. People with ADD can become so consumed by the complexity of getting everything done, that they do nothing. (p. 77) Magination Press, New York, 1994

Tip #7: Remembering info—write it down

A trick I learned in high school when studying French and Latin was that if I wrote the dialogue exercise down in long hand, I actually remembered it. Something about writing stuff down helps positively reinforce the retention.

Diane Y. Green

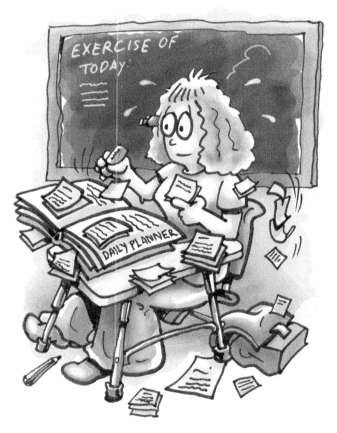

Tip #8: Retaining info—use color

Long before I realized I had AD/HD, I found that in my college years, highlighting books while reading helped me to retain the information. Also, color code your notebooks to match your school books, by subject. Remember too, that if you have documented that you have AD/HD and it impedes on your college success, you are entitled to receive school support. Head over to the college's student support office and discuss accommodations such as:

- Note takers
- Test taking in a quiet room
- Tape recording lectures
- Use of calculators
- Written directions provided by professor or student helper
- Extended time for test taking....and more

Terry Matlen

Chapter 8

A Hard Day's Night:
Thriving on the Job

AD/HD travels with us where ever we go from home to school to the workplace. We all want to excel in what we do for a living, yet our difficulty with focus and organization can, in some cases, cost us our jobs or at least that promotion we so earnestly desire and deserve. These tips can help make work life more pleasant and productive, helping us to meet and beat both our own expectations and those of our bosses. And if we can get away without asking for accommodations by coming up with our own—more power to us!

Careers

Tip #1: Finding a good fit—leave work at the office

Work in a field that allows you to leave your work at work. For instance, I am a nurse and when I leave for the day I do not have to worry about tons of paperwork to organize. When I am at work, I work "in the moment;" my ability to be creative and to be in touch with feelings and to my senses (sometimes being oversensitive) allows me to pick up on things going on with the patients I care for. Although being organized is a plus for nurses, nowadays there is so much struc-

ture built in to my profession that when I go home I
miss the structure I have at work.

Sabrina G.

Tip #2: Finding a good fit—look for variety
As far as work goes, I believe I have the perfect job
for being a woman with AD/HD. I am a dispatcher
for a food distribution company, and I am constantly
busy and always doing different things at work. In
any job to do with travel, dispatching, trucking, etc.,
the job is never the same from day to day. I also create my own to-do list at work for every day little things
I might forget and check them off as I go along. I
keep it where I can *see* it, so I don't forget I made a
list! Also, be patient with yourself. I had to learn that,
and it's hard.

Linda Baldomar-Moore
Anaheim, CA

Tip from Terry
In her book *Finding a Career That Works for
You,* Wilma Fellman offers these tips:
• Meet with your supervisor more frequently
  for feedback
• Have clear guidelines written for job perfor-
  mance
• Request training in time management skills
• Use checklists to determine job priorities and
  set deadline dates
• Ask for clerical help for paperwork (p. 91)

Reminders

Tip #3: Work—email reminders

Let's face it. I usually leave the office 20 to 30 minutes later than I have planned because I have to get just one more thing done: either deadlines are approaching or I think it will only take a second. However, I get charged $1 per minute for being late to daycare. Since I do not know what color my desk is because I have not seen it for months due to all the files I work on at once, I have resorted to emailing myself either a half-finished Word document or a note to remind myself of what I was doing when I had to rush off. This has saved a lot of time searching through the mass of paperwork to remember where I was and what I had done and what needs to be done next. I have found that this works a lot better than the task list reminders since I just ignore them.

Marilyn Hochman
Oviedo, FL

Tip #4: Remembering details—use Microsoft Outlook

I use Microsoft Outlook tasks tool. I put all my reminders in it so I do not have to remember anything—the less on my mind the better. I set the task to remind me of what I need to have done before they are due. It works best for me because I don't have to go to a day timer or calendar. I just have to make sure I leave Outlook open, and it will automatically remind me.

Juanita K Wilkins
Houston, TX

Tip #5: Staying on task—free software

There are lots of software programs that help you stay on task, but I found one that's simple to use, and it's free. It's just a little "To-Do" list that sits on your desktop:http://fp.futuresights.com/~angstrom/ todolist.html

Terry Matlen

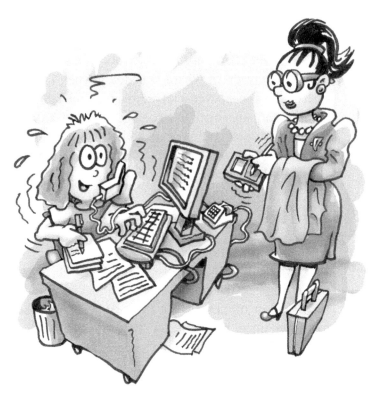

Organizing Tasks

Tip #6: Setting goals—To Do list

As far as getting stuff done at work, I find it very helpful to come up with a list of goals for the next day the evening before. That way when I come into work I simply follow the list until I get through it. Of course, I can't always finish everything on my list, but because I work in a very unstructured environment, I find it incredibly helpful so that I don't spend half of the morning trying to figure out what I am supposed to do!!!

Emily
San Francisco, CA

Tip #7: Recalling important info—use color

I am a math teacher and in my plans I used a color code system to alert my eyes to actually *read* my plans and recall important information: red means I need to give a quiz or test, green means I need to collect/check homework, blue means I need to collect/check projects or labs, and orange means class work.

Maykah M.

Minimizing Distractions

Tip #8: Being scattered—do one thing at a time

Once I get into something, I really cannot start anything else or I get all scattered. I know that the way I work best is to really only work on one thing at a time. For example, as a graduate student I could either do hands-on research or reading papers/writing papers. I found it incredibly hard to do both at the same time so I allowed myself weeks designated to reading and weeks designated to research. That way I could really get into something. Although this is not what my boss wants, I know for myself that this is the only way I can get the maximum amount of work done well.

Emily
San Francisco, CA

Tip #9: Focusing—add variety

I find that when I am at work, I have a lot of trouble concentrating on certain jobs for a long time. It is a lot easier now that I am on the meds, but I make sure that I vary my duties throughout the day. I work in an office so I might do filing for an hour, then do some typing, then follow up on some paperwork, and then go back to the filing. I just find that the variety makes it easier for me to get things accomplished. It helps that my boss is very understanding as her son also has AD/HD.

Rebecca Petrass
Canberra, Australia

Tip #10: Accomodating your AD/HD—various tips

Some do best sticking to one task till it's done; others need variety. Note what your working style is and go with your strengths. Note, too, that many of the accommodations I listed in the previous chapter can also be helpful at your place of work.
Some additional ones are:
- Requesting a quiet area to work in
- Allowing for work to be taken home, if possible
- Wearing headphones to block out noise
- Using written instructions, charts, and other visuals for assignments
- Taking frequent breaks

The ADA (Americans with Disabilities Act) protects you, but it can be tricky. Knowing if and when to disclose your AD/HD is beyond the scope of this book. I suggest you read up on the topic if you are having difficulties in this area. Refer to the Resources chapter at the end of this book.

Terry Matlen

Tip #11: Dealing with noise—white noise

To drown out distracting noise during the day at work, use a sound machine that plays white noise.

Cathlin Darling-Owen
Dummerston, VT

Tip #12: Focusing—go in early or stay late

I find it helpful to either get to work really early when no one is there yet because there are then fewer distractions or to come in a lot later in the day and then stay after everyone else has left.

Emily
San Francisco, CA

Scheduling

Tip #13: Scheduling—color coding work days

I work four days on and four days off, so I use highlighters to mark the days I work. If it's pink, I know I work that day. If its overtime, I mark that in pink and the time (payday is green). The days I teach are orange, etc. I'm very visual. The only problem is that the day planner I use is an all-year calendar and it starts in August. It's a college calendar year!

Jamie Placito
Syracuse, NY

Clutter

Tip #14: Paperwork sprawl—downsize your desk!

I was constantly getting overwhelmed at my big desk. A friend pointed out that I might not be so overwhelmed or disorganized if I had a smaller desk. I traded desks with a friend who had a small children's study desk and I *love* it. My desk is just the right size for my computer and to write short notes but too small for piles of papers. Since there is no space, I find myself using my filing cabinet or just throwing things away, plus there is less on the desk to distract me while I work. All I have on the desk is the computer, a pad of paper and a pen, and my timer to keep me on track.

Joan Tattum
Philadelphia, PA

General Tips

Tip #15: Overall issues—various tips

- Know your energy patterns: Try to maximize your peak hours of clear focus.
- Do *more* than you need to when you are particularly "on target."
- Work with a coach (behind the scenes) to set up a clean, efficient, organized work space.
- Be mindful of colors, textures, scents, sounds, and other environmental elements that might affect you in the workplace.
- Keep your work wardrobe simple to cut down on "wardrobe malfunction" distractions!
- Find music that motivates you but doesn't distract you.
- Block off peak hours of focus for work tasks, and when working at home, be sure family

interference are limited to emergencies.

- Feel "put together" in your professional appearance. We tend to perform better professionally when we look and feel professional. (Work with an image consultant or a free one in a store near you.)
- Leave some "start up" and "summary" time at the start and end of each day to pull any loose ends together.

Wilma Fellman, M.Ed., L.P.C.
Career counselor specializing in AD/HD
W. Bloomfield, MI

Chapter 9

Any Time at All:
Time and Data Management

For us women with AD/HD, time seems to have a life of its own—it stretches into weird configurations, pops up intrusively with its rude little buzzers and beepers, and generally puts a crimp in our style. Women with AD/HD truly do have a different experience of time than most: an hour can seem like a minute and vice-versa. Like trying to lasso Jello, time is elusive, slippery, and ever-changing in its form—and a *constant* source of frustration. Is it possible to end our never-ending quarrels with time? Or at least develop a relationship based on respect even if love is out of the question? Definitely!

In addition to our struggles with managing time, we also suffer from the relentless barrage of infinitesimal bits of data coming at us like enemy fire. How can we keep from getting totally annihilated? Weapons! Highly specialized tactical weapons called PDAs, planners, organizers, and calendars. Run, don't walk, to your nearby office supply store and stock up today! Buying such high-class weapons won't take away all of our time management problems, but they sure will help. And the tips that follow will give you expert advice on how to use them most effectively.

Data Management

Tip #1: Scheduling—color coding family members

I write everyone's appointments, sporting events, etc., in my planner and then use different color highlighters for each person. For example, I'm pink, my husband is green, my oldest son is yellow, and my youngest is blue. You could also do this just by using different color pens, of course, but I find the "neon" effect from the highlighters really helps me.

Sheila S.
Norwalk, OH

Tip #2: Data management and organizing tasks—colored notepad

I bought a notepad from the grocery store that has four colors of paper: red, yellow, green, and purple. I write a master list on the purple, put it in my appointment book, and keep it with me all the time. I write down what I *want* to do on the green pages, what I *have* to do on the yellow pages (particularly things that have a deadline and or involve a promise or obligation to someone else), and use the red pages like a *red alert*!!!! Anything on that list is something that needs immediate attention. Each week I move things around on my pages; red list items are priority and new things go on my green/fun and yellow/must-do lists. Sometimes I also wear red jewelry or a red t-shirt to remind me I'm doing red items that day. I may not be able to finish all of a project, but I do all that *I* can.

Once I'm done with a project from any colored page, I put a gold star on my calendar page. I also make certain I do at least one green-page fun task a week as a reward to keep balance in my life. Since I started my color-coded pages, I've not had to medicate at all. The colors made all the difference in turning my world from a rainy, depressed, unproductive day to a day filled with rainbow colors and gold stars!

Rose Heath
Birmingham, AL

Tip #3: Data management—three-ring binders

I use three-ring binders for each child and immediately file report cards, IEPs, evaluations, etc., in different sections of the binder so I have everything all in one place. I have a section with notebook paper and I document any calls to teachers, counselors, etc., so I also have a record of who I called, why, when, and what the result was. I also keep track of concerns or relevant articles I have that I want to bring up at meetings that might support what I'm saying. Then when it's time for IEP meetings, all I have to do is grab each child's binder, and I have everything I need. Everyone is so impressed with how organized I am. Hah! If they only knew! I have ADD, my eleven-year-old child has AD/HD and mild Autism, and my eight-year-old child has a speech delay and gets OT.

Sheila S.
Norwalk, OH

Planners

Tip #4: Being late—build in extra time

Since I am consistently late to appointments (and consistently embarrassed by that), I have begun writing the appointment time one half hour earlier than the real scheduled appointment time and then treat it as if

99

it is the actual appointment time. I get to be on time and it feels really good for a change. Also, at the time I am rescheduling, I have my calendar out and write my next appointment in it. Receptionists used to give me little cards with the next appointment date and time, but I would always lose them.

Michaela
Salem, OR

Tip #5: Organizing systems—master list on planner cards
You know the Franklin Covey planners? I use their plastic pouch page-finder/ruler and the back (the note side) of the "weekly compass" cards to keep my master task list. I try to put my "to do" stuff on that task list and then keep moving the plastic piece to the current day. That way my list is always in front of me, and I take the planner with me everywhere. I try to pick at least five things from the list each day. (You can find it at: www.myADDstore.com)

Mandy Ronaldson
Sacramento, CA

Tip #6: Saving money on planners—try three-ring binders
I got a small (9" x 7") three-ring binder at an office supply place. It's cheaper than a brand name calendar/planner, and I found one with a clear plastic cover (Avery, View Binder). I personalized it with a beautiful greeting card (which could be changed seasonally if I had the time!) The local dime store sells small (8 _" x 5 _") pages of three-ring notebook style paper for notes, etc. I purchase calendar pages that give me one month on two pages. When my book is opened, I can see the whole month, which helps with planning.

A few brand name calendars (e.g., Daytimer, Franklin Covey) fit perfectly. The store bought calendars are worth the money; the paper is stronger than if you printed it out yourself on your computer. The calendars come in a couple of styles, and they are tabbed to find easily in a notebook.

Donna R.N
Encinitas, CA

Capturing Ideas

Tip #7: Capturing ideas—notebook

I have helped myself a lot by purchasing a small notebook and carrying it in my purse. When I think of something that I need to do, or if I need to buy something or if someone gives me information, I just jot it down in my book. Then I do not have to search or try to remember information that I know I will forget.

GW

Tip #8: Capturing ideas—notes in pocket

If I'm not home, and I want to remember something, I write a small note on a very small piece of paper and put it in my pants pocket. When I take the pants off at night, it becomes automatic (most of the time) to check the pockets for the note, and if not, I remember before washing them to look for the note. I also know where a phone number might be if I use this method. If this isn't possible, I use the answering machine method.

Cathlin Darling-Owen
Dummerston, VT

Tip #9: Capturing ideas—make lists
> Make lists and post them in a conspicuous place like the refrigerator or even the mirror in the bathroom. I've used Post-its and put them on the rear view mirror in my car or on the outside of my purse.
>
> Tamara Gabrielsen
> Halsey, OR

Tip #10: Capturing ideas—use answering machine and Post-its
> I will often call my own answering machine and leave myself a message at home or work. Good places for Post-it note reminders are on my computer screen, on the bathroom mirror, over the speedometer on my car dash, or on the TV screen for my son after school.
>
> Laura Tobin
> Woodstock, IL

Tip #11: Capturing ideas—magnetic board
> I think it is helpful to have a magnetic board on the fridge, one of those erasable ones. I make a list, (a realistic one!) so that I can check items off after doing them. I feel better about myself when I have done things as opposed to doing nothing and laying around.
>
> Laura Oleson
> Howard Lake, MN

Tip #12: Capturing ideas—three-ring binders
> Get one of those three ring binders that zips closed and use that for all of your daily planning and any

papers you need to keep with you. I sewed a long strap to mine and carry it on my shoulder like a purse. Now it works great.

Wendy Wolfington
College Station, TX

Tip #13: Capturing ideas—notepad in car

I have a pen on a string from the dollar store. I have taken cheap notepads and used a hole punch and put them in the car. I even tied it to the car. This worked until my husband cleaned the car and removed it once. I was lost for months without it. I get a lot of my thoughts while driving the kids places. Of course now he knows not to do that again.

Cathlin Darling-Owen
Dummerston, VT

Tip #14: Reducing accumulation of little notes—use notebooks

I have a tendency (and don't most of you?) to jot down phone messages, ideas, plans, etc. on little scraps of paper that end up in scary piles all over the house. To solve this problem, I've used the following system:

- Keep one major notebook for important notes and leave it in your main work area, e.g., home office. When you get a call or need to keep information handy, write it *all* down there, no exceptions.
- Keep Post-it pads by every phone in your house. Jot down your messages there, then either transpose them into your main notebook

or just stick them onto the page. Always, always…date each page in your book.

Terry Matlen

Timers

Tip #15: Time management—countdown timers

What saved my sanity the most while my kids were growing up was having a watch with a countdown-timer that could also be set to beep on the hour. Some people find it annoying to have their watch beep every 60 minutes, but it really helped pull me back into time instead of "space." I could lock into whatever I was doing without the diversion of trying to remember what time it was. The same with the countdown timer…15 minutes to pick up a room, maybe get on the Internet for a couple of minutes and still leave for an appointment on time or go back and put the spaghetti in the water for supper before the water evaporated. This has worked pretty good for "time outs," too. This was a really inexpensive watch and so easy to use. Just click a button for 1, 5, 10, 20, 30-minute increments. Many of the other watches, when you can find such a feature, I found just too tedious to set. (You can find watches that beep at www.myADDstore.com)

Sophia Lahen
New Hampshire

Tip #16: Time management—timer for everything

I use a timer for everything and make a project fun. For example, every morning I pick a random time such as 14 minutes and 13 seconds and set the timer. I put on up-beat music and get whatever cleaning/straightening done as fast as I can. When the timer goes off,

I stop. It is fun to beat the clock *and* have a clean living environment!

Deborah D.

Tip #17: Departure times—do a countdown
I have timers placed around the house. I use them so I know how much time I have left before I have to leave. Of course, in this family, I have to add in extra time. If I add in too much time, we'll be late for sure.

Cathlin Darling-Owen
Dummerston, VT

General Time Management Advice
Tip #18: Prioritizing—rate your tasks

How to prioritize:

1. List the tasks which need to be completed.
2. Assign an "importance value" to each, using the scale 1-4 (1 is most important, 4 is least important).
3. Ask "How important is it for me to do this task?" Write it down.
4. Assign an "urgency value" as above. "How *soon* must this task be completed?"
5. Calculate a total by multiplying the two values together.
6. Rewrite the list according to the new values assigned to each task, starting with 1.

Deborah Lancaster
Sunnyvale, CA
(Note: See appendix for Deborah's prioritizing chart.)

Tip #19: Time management—prioritizing

I have to write down all of the tasks that I would like to accomplish for the day. Then I prioritize the top three to five. I may do an easy one first to feel that I have accomplished something. If I am dreading one, I do it first to get if off my mind. Tasks that are not completed are moved to the next day's list if I still need to finish them. A new list is created and so it goes. Without my list I rarely accomplish anything that I don't want to do.

Maureen

Tip #20: Being on time—set clocks ahead

To be on time (I tell people this is from my twisted blonde logic), I set all of the clocks in my house, my wristwatches, and the clock in my car 15 minutes ahead. Time savers for getting ready in the morning: choose your clothes, shoes, and accessories the night before and set them out. Realistically figure out how much time it takes to get ready to leave the house.

Tamara Gabrielsen
Halsey, OR

Tip #21: Time management for personal hygiene—rubber boots

Since I can't sit still (the joke is that I get in and out of the bathtub three times before I ever get wet), I pour an inch of water into an old pair of rain boots to soak my feet. Then I can slosh around and do chores and not have to stay in one place for the half hour or so it takes to soften me up for a pedicure.

Carole Read
Santa Rosa, California

Tip #22: Keeping track of time—alarms

I have a palm pilot with alarms, and my son has a *Watch-Minder* watch that has been successful for him. I lose track of time when I am on my lunch hour or in a store, so I have a watch with a timer and set it as I leave for lunch. I give myself a five or ten minute warning so I get back to work on time.

Laura Tobin
Woodstock, IL

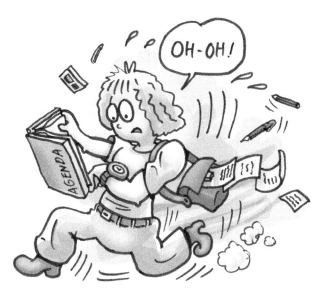

Tip #23: Efficient use of time for errands—choose providers by location, location, location!!

I select otherwise comparable service providers based on their proximity to my home and/or office. For instance, my dry cleaner is located halfway between my home and office in a shopping center where there is

also a house wares store that I like. I do the same
with the auto repair shop, movie rental store, hairstyl-
ist, and even the babysitter!

Karen F.

*Tip #24: Finding time to get paperwork done—double up
with fun stuff*

I hate paper work but find that I can get things like
that done while doing other, more pleasant things like
watching TV. Combine things you hate to do with
things you enjoy. Or take it with you to places like
doctor's appointments, hairdressers...so you can get
them done while you're waiting.

Mikki Conners
Chicago, IL

Tip #25: Overbooking—just say "No!"

We like to please; we seem to *need* to please and that's
why we haven't learned to say "No." When you're
asked to bake brownies for the kids' Girl Scout meeting or upcoming church fundraiser, learn to say "Let
me think about it and get back to you." Then go home
and ask yourself if you really have time to do it. If
the answer is no, call the person and apologize but
offer to help out another time in the future. You'll be
amazed at how easy this becomes with time.

Terry Matlen

Tip #26: Getting it all done—work with your strengths

I'm a morning person by my husband is a night owl.
We use this to our advantage; I can get the kids'

lunches packed in the AM, and he helps the kids with their homework in the evening. The point is to know what your internal clock is and go with it.

Layne Carlyle
Stratford, Ontario
Canada

Chapter 10

We Can Work it Out:
Relationships and Social Skills

Poor self-esteem, difficulty with self-reflection, and lack of social skills can make it difficult for us to maintain strong relationships. Those ancient voices in our heads—memories of past failures and criticisms from parents and teachers—stay with us like ghosts, creeping in daily to undermine our self-confidence. Too often we have embarrassed ourselves with the impulsive word blurted out without pause to reflect on its potential impact, thus creating distance and anxiety both with our nearest and dearest as well as with new acquaintances. Throw in the fact that we often don't have the *energy* to make things work, and we can see why relationships present such a challenge to women with AD/HD. Read on to see how others have found ways to improve relationships in their lives.

General Advice

Tip #1: Sorting out the important stuff—lighten up

Don't take yourself too seriously. Just because you feel something is a major disaster that must be sorted out now doesn't mean that you have to go in with big lead boots. Phone a friend or ask advice if you are unsure.

Tanya Billings
London, England, UK

Tip #2: Handling disagreements—open door policy

I have an open door policy. If you disagree with me, I figure I'm an adult, and we can have differences. My kids are not afraid to come to me about anything. I may just need a cool down period. But they are allowed cool down periods, too, which helps prevent screaming and saying things you do not mean and can never take back.

Cherity Kingston
Wilcox, NE

Tip #3: Change in friendships—letting go

Let it be okay that some friends have to be dropped because they don't reciprocate and/or aren't good for your mental or emotional health.

Donna Parten
Sacramento, CA

Support

Tip #4: Finding support—use your friends and pets

Have at least one (preferably more) friends you can really be yourself with that *know* your impairments and can help you stay on track. I think women especially need that support. Family is not always the best place to "open up," and women need a place to "blurt," bounce, express intense feelings, etc. without feeling threatened. We need that unconditional acceptance of who we are. Animals help, too! Get a pet. If you can't, sit others' pets and take frequent zoo trips!

Sharon V. Galloway
Wilmington, NC

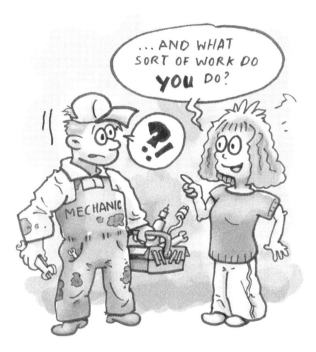

Communication Skills

Tip #5: Communication skills—various tips

Mentally remind yourself to wait your turn to speak. Maintain eye contact with the speaker(s). Remember to ask people how they are and what their thoughts are. Other people want to communicate, too. Take communications classes. Remember you aren't going to remember much from seminars that last for several hours. I recommend classes of longer duration on-line or at the local community college.

Tamara Gabrielsen
Halsey, OR

Tip #6: Being assertive—take classes

I have found that taking an assertiveness training class really helped me. Just learning how to talk to non-ADD people without becoming aggressive or staying passive has made a world of difference in my life.

Claudia Teague

Tip #7: Maintaining self-esteem—train others how to speak to you

Another thing that I do that might help you is to correct people when they ask you, "What did you *do* today?" I absolutely *hate* that. I might not have *done* anything measurable to speak of, but I may have thought, planned, designed a way to be more effective, struggled to keep on track, etc. I focus on the time issue, not the quantity of tasks I perform or the importance or impact of my task or project. I only focus on whether I've started a project, whether I'm on track with it, and celebrate the completion of it.

Rose Heath
Birmingham, AL

Tip #8: Finding time to talk—emails

I recommend communicating with your spouse through emails if you have a difficult time communicating. I usually will type an email when I am angry, then save it as a draft. Once I have calmed down, either later that day or sometime during the week, I will go back and reread it. If I still feel it is appropriate to send, I will do so. Most of the time, I don't send it, I just use it to spout off.

Laura Oleson
Howard Lake, MN

Tip #9: Dealing with distractions—no TV
When having a conversation of any substance, do it in a room with no TV. Also, use "I" statements versus "You do this..." "Why don't you see how it makes *me* feel...?" If we understand how other look at things, I think it makes better us realize how we affect people.

Jamie Placito
Syracuse, NY

Tip #10: Softening the "No"—alternatives
I saw a list in a women's magazine once of various ways to say no when just saying a plain no doesn't feel right or is too hard to do. When you say no in these ways, you don't have to explain the real reasons, but you can make it sound better than a plain no, if you need to do that to feel better.

- "NO, not this year"
- "I've done it before, and I'll do it again but not right now."
- "No, but thanks for asking. That makes me feel good."
- "No, I'm involved in too much right now."
- "You know, I really believe in that project, but I wouldn't be able to give it my full attention right now."

- If all else fails, "No, probably not, but I'll check with ___ and see if it is possible to fit it in."

I've been on the asking side, and I keep two things in mind: Asking someone to do something means that I have confidence that that person can do the job, which can be seen as empowering or a compliment. Secondly, I appreciate a sincere no much more than a yes from someone who doesn't follow through. So be honest if you can't give a good effort to something at the moment. What are your priorities right now? Does this fit in at this point in time?

Lois Garbisch
Cook, MN

Tip #11: Effective listening—reflecting back the message
Repeat what other people are telling you; it's courteous and maintains accuracy and so is appreciated more than not; it also helps to get it into the working memory, which is most important.

Mary B.

Tip #12: Shyness—ask about them

Are you at a loss for words in social situations? Shy? Afraid you'll fumble? People *love* to talk about themselves, in general, so ask, ask, ask about their lives, kids, work, hobbies, etc. With time, you will begin to feel more confident so that you can talk more about *yourself*, too. Compliments and praise go a long way, too.

Terry Matlen

Tip #13: Keeping the peace at home—weekly pow-wows
I want my husband to realize that many of the things I

116

do—or don't do—are related to my ADD and are not intentional behaviors on my part. We try and have weekly meetings to go over the things I do that aggravate him (and vice versa!) and come up with game plans. If he knows I will most likely forget to buy his favorite foods at the market, we talk about ways to remind me without his making me feel worse than I already do. Marital therapy helped a *lot,* and I'd recommend it, especially with someone who really understands how the ADD affects relationships.

Anna Ramsey
Boulder, CO

Note from Terry

Dr. Michele Novotni talks extensively about AD/HD adults and Social Skills in her book, "What Does Everyone Know That I Don't?" Here's one gem on how to enter a conversation:

"It's... best to listen to the conversation for a bit before jumping in. Try to understand what they're talking about so you don't disrupt the flow of the conversation" (p. 138).

She also notes how, in conversations, adults with AD/HD worry about forgetting their thoughts and thus often interrupt to get their words out before they're lost. She suggests evaluating how important those words are for that moment, and if they can wait, to jot them down on a piece of paper.

Chapter 11

Come Together:
Parenting and Family

As women, we share the social burden of being expected to do it all: super mom, super lover, super worker, and super socialite. As women with AD/HD, we have the added burden of trying to do it all without adequate tools. Imagine being asked to build a house and instead of having a nifty little red tool box and a cool leather tool belt, all of your tools are buried under boards and scattered about in piles, nails and all. And half of your workers have the same problem! The chances of a woman with AD/HD having children with AD/HD is approximately 50%. How do other women with AD/HD cope with such challenges?

Behavior and Discipline
Tip #1: Motivation—rewards

> The only way I can get my daughter to be on time in the morning is to make her a chart that she checks off showing the order of things to do. When Friday comes, if 90% of her chart is marked and she has had good behavior, she gets to go to the treasure box and pick one thing, like dollar store stuff, or coupons good

for staying up late, dinner of her choice, movie etc. It has worked wonders for her being on time and behaving.

GW

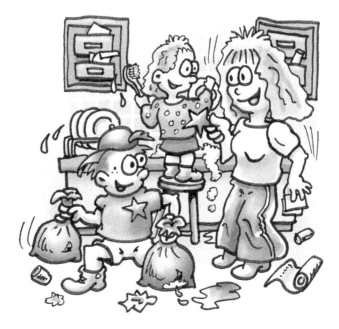

Tip #2: Motivating—use popcorn

I took a tip from my old fourth-grade teacher, Mrs. Forrest, who did a really neat thing to get our cooperation. I have a clear plastic cup taped to a piece of paper and stuck on the fridge. The cup has a black line drawn on it. I got some popcorn kernels and told my kids, "Whenever I catch you being good, I will give you kernels to put in the cup. When it reaches the line, we will have a popcorn party, rent a movie, and have a friend over." They earn popcorn for doing things the first time I ask, for picking up after themselves, for being nice to each other... just any little thing. It pumps up their ego, encourages good behavior, and when they see their siblings earning popcorn, they hurry up and get on the ball to earn some too! It's easier for me than trying to remember sticker charts or poker chips. And they earn them when they *don't* ask me for them. So that eliminates them bugging me for it.

Sandy
Attica, IN

Tip #3: Quarreling between siblings—give it back to them
As a single AD/HD parent with two AD/HD boys, I was always trying to get one of us on track! Two of my worst nemeses were the daily responsibilities and chores and the eternal argument of who sits in the front seat of the car. Here were the remedies that worked like a charm but *only* if you set the rules in stone and *never* deviate from them. The best part for me is that it took me completely out of two struggles that had previously been the bane of my life. They work!

Chores: Together we created a schedule of each of their chores and responsibilities on a daily check sheet and posted it in the kitchen. Then I explained to them that all privileges and permissions would be granted predicated on that check list remaining up to date. After that, when they would ask for permission to do things (within our families set limits of course), I would turn the question around to them and say, "I don't know. You tell me, can you? What does the chart show?" Well, this caught on like a charm. They enjoyed the control over their own destiny and having that written schedule was very helpful to them as a reminder and a way to check themselves!

Front Seat: I assigned them each odds and evens based on there birthdates (this, of course, could be adjusted to anything that will determine odds and evens.) Each time we rode in the car, whatever the date was, odds or even, that's the one who would sit in the front that entire day. This stopped all the fighting instantly and forever!

June Michaels
San Francisco, CA

Tip #4: Rewarding good behavior—shredding
Kids *love* to shred. Involve them in this process; maybe even use it as a reward for good behaviors.

Ally Reinhart
Concord, MA

Tip #5: Stop the nagging—make them hold their agreements in their hands
Often ADD kids have ADD moms. We remember to tell our kids to do something, and they, of course, are in the middle of a TV show. "I'll do it at the commercial" is commonly heard. Of course, by the time the commercial comes on we have both forgotten the chore until sometime later when we remember and the same game begins again. One way to solve this dilemma is to have Post-it notes handy or even large pieces of laminated cardboard. Write the request on the Post-it or cardboard such as "Bring laundry upstairs" or "Take trash out." The child must hold the

piece of paper until they do the chore at the next commercial. If they put it down, the TV goes off immediately. I have found that most often the child gets up and does the chore when the commercial comes on because the paper is annoying to hold and serves as a constant reminder of the agreement.

Jeri Goldstein, R.N., MC
Phoenix, AZ

Traveling with Kids

Tip #6: Reduce the nagging—involve them with a calendar
One trick I use with my children is when they ask me how many nights I am going to be gone when traveling. I say, for example, "Four sleep nights." Then I give them a calendar and they mark off the sleep nights.

Tip #7: Keeping kids entertained—scavenger hunt
When we went on vacation in Florida, I gave each kiddo a list of things they had to look for (kind of like a scavenger hunt) and some things they had to get, like a napkin with the name of the restaurant in which they ate—all kinds of things. Then we would check the list each night. The one that found the most got to choose a dessert or would get to choose from the "surprise bag" first. For each trip I made the scavenger hunt geared toward what we were going to be doing. For example, this weekend we are going to see the Reds play, so I thought of making a list of things that are red that they have to find. It's a lot of family fun, plus they are learning, and they don't even know it.

Karen S. Fox
Louisville, KY

Sleep

Tip #8: Restlessness at night—try a fish tank

We started with fish tanks originally to help my son sleep. The tank was his night light, and he could occupy his mind and relax watching the fish, whereas a book or TV would keep his mind awake and stimulated until the story ended.

Laura Tobin
Woodstock, IL

Tip #9: Winding down—lavender oil

To help hyperactive children settle down in the evening, burn lavender essential oil. If they are particularly hyped up, try putting some on their mattress or under their pillow. I have four AD/HD children and have been using this successfully for years.

S. Wilton
Tara Qld, Australia

Minimizing Distractions

Tip #10: Dealing with distractions—creating special space

My son is eight-years old and has AD/HD. For homework time, my son goes to a very quiet place away from everyone else. If that isn't possible, we have tried letting him listen to soft music (no words) on a headset. At school he gets very bothered by the noise from the other students, so his teacher moved him to a desk closer to hers (away from the window), and it has dividers on both sides so he isn't as distracted.

For behavior, we have a chart on the fridge with categories like not being rude from wake up time until school time, not fighting with brothers during lunch time, etc. He gains points for good behavior and gets a reward at the end of the day or week depending on how many points he has. I also try to give him "special time," this is one-on-one time without the other kids, at least 20 minutes twice a week. He seems to need a lot more good attention than his brothers do. Special time is anything he picks such as a board game with mom or a visit to the park with dad. Parenting a child with AD/HD is very hard most of the time, but the more praise I give him for being good, the easier it is for us to get along, and the better he feels about himself instead of always getting into trouble for being *bad*!

Pam
Ontario, Canada

Tip #11: Building up self-esteem—more praise

Children with AD/HD are bombarded with negative comments and demands. This does a real number on their self-esteem. Try counting how many times in one day you reprimand, yell, correct, direct, and discipline your child. Now count how many times you praise in that same time frame, and you may be shocked. This was a huge wakeup call for me with my own AD/HD daughter. Remember to "catch them being good" and express your delight. This goes a long way in building their self-esteem.

Terry Matlen

Tip #12: Overwhelming them—ask for feedback

I tell my son to let me know when I am asking him to do too many things at a time (or jumping from one thing to another, or deciding to go for burgers and changing to pizza half way through and coming back to burgers.) My son is my little "police officer." I also stop many times during the day to think about what I am going to say to him and how, so I do not drive him crazy. I do rehearse!

Maykah M.

Chores

Tip #13: Motivating them—use a timer

If I have children doing chores, I pick a chore, and they pick a chore, I set a timer for a certain amount of time, and we do not leave that room or that chore until the timer has gone off. Then they cannot play or do something that they want to do until the chore is completed, or the timer goes off.

Karen Roberts
Yuma, Arizona

Tip #14: Motivating them—let them choose

My ADD kids, like many, hated *hated* being told what to do, especially in the arena of taking care of their chores. What worked for me was to, instead of giving directives, give them a choice between two chores: "Would you like to pick up your books or help me take out the garbage"?

Hannah McArthur
Casper, Wyoming

Balancing Family Time with Self-regeneration

Tip #15: Revolving door family—take shifts

I had to give up the perfect picture of our family sitting down together every night for dinner. We have three young children, and by the time my husband walks in the door at night, I am ready to walk out. So that's what we do. They have a couple of hours of solo time with Daddy; I grab some physical and mental space and make it back to read books before bedtime. This makes it possible for me to have anything left to share with my spouse later in the evening. The hardest part is letting go of the guilt. I keep reminding myself that I am lousy as a short order cook but fabulous at cuddling on the couch and sharing stories.

Trish
Wisconsin

Connecting

Tip #16: Spacing out—use an agreed upon trigger to bring you back

How can you stay connected when you regularly space out and daydream? By being aware of your tendency towards distraction and daydreaming, you can discuss with your children ways for them to pull you back in, explaining to them that your behavior at such times is not intentional, reassuring them of your love and interest, but perhaps developing a signal that the family can use to help reconnect. One idea could be a "trigger" comment (not meant to criticize or be-little mom) like "Earth to mom!" You need to continually self-monitor, too, and take notice of your tendencies, making special efforts to connect with your children. Medications for AD/HD are extremely helpful in keeping one "in the moment", thereby helping you to stay focused. Children and spouses need frequent reminders that they are loved and appreciated. Set aside special one-on-one time with each child, letting the child take the lead in fun activities. Dr. Stanley Greenspan, a gifted psychiatrist and author, discusses "floor time," which are child-lead activities to help parents and their children connect emotionally.

Terry Matlen

Tip #17: Feeling overwhelmed—get a sitter even when you're home

It's imperative that AD/HD moms find ways to help themselves in the often overwhelming situation of trying to raise one or more AD/HD children. I often suggest bringing in babysitters *even when mom is home* so that she can have another set of hands to help with the children. High-school or college students are wonderful support systems; they have the energy to keep up with the often hyperactive children, especially if mom has the inattentive subtype of AD/HD and is easily overwhelmed in such an active household.

In my own case, I've utilized sitters to help me with my own AD/HD daughter and have been blessed with women who not only love her high energy but who also have been able to help me organize her mountains of belongings, clothes, etc.

Tanya Eckberg
Braintree, MA

Tip #18: Mealtime mania—be flexible

I have two AD/*HHHH*D (extremely hyperactive!) kids who can't sit still at meal time. I thought for sure I was going to develop ulcers from all the ruckus and from me shouting at them day at breakfast, lunch, and dinner. Then I realized that there was no golden rule that said they have to sit in their chairs at every meal. So when they are particularly unsettled, I let them eat standing up or even sprawled out on two chairs. Sometimes I let them eat in another room in front of the TV (I've found that the distraction of the TV gets them to eat more than they normally do). Now mealtimes are *much* more relaxing for all of us. I only hope their future wives don't kill me.

Sandrine Willems
Brussels, Belgium

Tip #19: Picky eaters—various tips

Mine are the pickiest eaters. No sandwiches allowed in their lunch boxes and anything green is evil. They are revolted if their foods touch on their plates. Here's how I've worked through this: For lunch, instead of the usual PB & J sandwiches that most children enjoy, I pack little samplers of things in various baggies. Here are some example ideas: small bits of cheese, mini bagel, or favorite fruit sliced in "odd" ways to lend interest. Once I was able to get my daughter to eat a jelly sandwich by removing the crust and cutting it out into fun shapes (faces were a hit); cheese sticks, cold pasta noodles with Parmesan cheese, etc. It's exhausting to come up with creative ideas all the time, but it does get them to eat better. To keep food from touching, I buy those plastic trays that have divided spaces. To get greens into them, I mash things like green beans and broccoli and sneak them into meatloaf, burgers, etc. They're also more likely to eat raw veggies if they can dip them in Ranch dressing.

Janice Danto
Portland, OR

Tip #20: Transition from work to home—take a break

After a full day at work, coming to a full house of ADD kids and a spouse, I *know* I need downtime before entering the ADD zone. I have ADD, too, and it's just too overwhelming to come home to such chaos, so I stop for a coffee break at Starbucks to recharge. I'm a much better mom when I come home, once I have had some down time. If I can't stop somewhere on the way home, I let my family know ahead of time that I need 15 minutes at home— *alone*—before going full swing into my mommy role. Sometimes that means retreating to the bathroom!

Shannon Selik
Savannah, GA

Tip #21: Re-charging your batteries—take much needed breaks

It is essential that AD/HD moms get away so they can re-charge. Let go of the guilt and remember that you need to take care of *you*, and by doing so, you'll have more patience with your kids, which more than likely includes one or more with AD/HD. Take weekends off at least four times a year, even if it means holing up at a nearby hotel. Allow yourself the bliss of sleeping in, catching up with your reading, or just vegging out in front of the TV. This is not a luxury; this is a necessity. Now go book a room!

Terry Matlen

Tip #22: Managing conflict—pick your battles

Pick your battles! I used to go head to head with my daughter over the stupidest things, like making sure she wore a sweatshirt under her coat. Sheesh! If she's cold, she'll put on something warm. Let it go and you'll both be happier.

Danielle Harris
Colorado Springs, CO

Tip #23: Homework battles—get a tutor

My son has AD/HD and learning disabilities. I hate to admit it, but I have *no patience* helping him with his daily homework. Both our meds wear off at the same time. As a single mom, I don't have anyone else in the house to help him, so I got smart and hired a high-school student who was looking for some extra cash and who was willing to come by a few days a week to help my son with his work. Our evenings are so much pleasanter now. The added bonus is that my son has a male role model that he can relate to. No more power struggles for us!

Tanya Richard
Mobile, AL

Note from Terry

Keep in mind that if you have children with AD/HD and it impacts on their academic success, then they are probably eligible for special school services under a 504 plan or an IEP.

> Visit Wright's Laws and Reed Martin's excel-
> lent Web sites for more information:
> www.wrightslaw.com
> www.reedmartin.com

> In his 1995 book, *Taking Charge of AD/HD*,
> Dr. Russell Barkley suggests setting up rules
> with your AD/HD children before entering a
> public place:
>
> Just before you enter a public place, stop
> and review the important rules of conduct
> with your child. Give your child about three
> rules that he or she commonly violates in
> that particular place and tell the child to say
> them back to you... (p. 170).

Tip #24: Managing excess energy—provide energy burners
Supply your child with plenty of opportunities to burn
off excessive energy. A small trampoline works great!
Giving him/her fidgets to use during school and homework also are great focusing tools. You can find many
at www.myADDstore.com

Terry Matlen

*Tip #25: Handling phone time—provide distractions and a
notepad*
It never fails. When I get a phone call, my little ADDer
wants my attention at that *same moment*. I keep a basket of coloring books and crayons near the phone to
keep her occupied. But sometimes I will resort to

hiding in my bedroom. I have a sign I hang from the doorknob: *Off Duty*. I leave a notebook on the floor so she can jot down a note instead of having to interrupt me.

Kimberly Gould
Virginia Beach, VA

Tip #26: Grocery shopping—use the avoidance tactic
This one is simple: Don't take them grocery shopping with you!

Heather Mansfield
Sheffield, UK

Tip #27: Grocery shopping—make it a game
This was always a nightmare for me until we started making a game of it. Now we have a scavenger hunt. I give each child a list of things I need, and the first one to find them earns a treat at the check out counter.

Marlene Greenhill
Fremont, CA

Tip# 28: Preventing tantrums—give gentle reminders
My ADDer doesn't transition well. At ten, he still tantrums when I tell him to get ready for bed while he's intently playing his Game Boy. What I found that works is giving him reminders starting 30 minutes before bedtime and continuing at intervals of 15, 10 then 5 minutes. This way, he doesn't seem so jolted from moving into the next phase of his day.

Susan Jansen
Fresno, CA

Chapter 12

Money:
Managing Finances

We say we'd pay our bills if only we had the money in the bank. Guess again! It's not always about how much we bring home but what we do with it once that check is in the bank (if it makes it to the bank!) The torture of staying on track, keeping our bills in one place, and then *remembering* to pay them on time is not an easy task. Here are some ideas to help keep your money working for you.

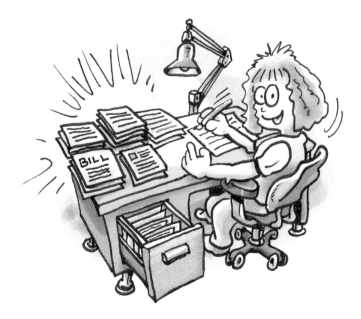

Paying Bills

Tip #1: Avoid late fees—use one credit card

I pay all bills on time, every time, by charging everything to one credit card and having that card on direct withdrawal from my checking account to be paid in full monthly. I keep the account balanced by looking at the top and bottom lines of the statement to make sure that what it says at the top is about the same as what it says at the bottom, i.e., the dollar amount I begin with each month is approximately the same as what I end with each month. My income is the same each month, so I make my outgoing expenses the same each month. I manage the outgoing expenses by using willpower. I don't do math, so this works well. If I need more money, I rent out bedrooms.

The Irish Cookie
Long Island, NY

Tip #2: Avoid late fees—use online banking

The best thing ever for paying bills on time is internet banking. The next best thing is marking the due dates a week early on the calendar. That way when you pay them on your highlighted date, it's good and early.

Angela S.
Quesnel, BC

Tip #3: Avoid late fees—use a service that pays bills for you!

I have found it is worth paying $11/month for what I'll refer to as ELITE online billpay. Certainly banks offer very useful bill paying services without charge, but you still have to remember to sign on and pay your bills on time! The company I have found (www.paytrust.com) allows me to set up a totally mindless system. My bills go directly to them. When a bill comes in, I get an email notice. I can login and pay it then or, if I ignore it, thinking I'll do it later, I get another email prior to the bill being paid late, to *really* log in then. Like most systems, you can set up recurring payments so you never have to think about them and can pay things that don't have an incoming bill. This is the one system that has eliminated my late fees!

Ellen
Charlotte, NC

Tip #4: Avoid late fees—use a master spreadsheet

I used to make late payments every month! My solution was to make a spreadsheet that lists all of my bills, the date received, the date due, the date sent, amount owed, amount paid, and check number. At the beginning of the year, I make a sheet for each month and print them out and place them into a three ring binder. Each day when I get home from work, I get the mail and the binder and start listing the bills I received that day, including the due date and the amount due. I then place all of the bills into a file cabinet folder labeled "Unpaid Bills" by due date. Every Saturday, I get my binder and my unpaid bills and pay the ones that are due within the next 10 days. It helps to keep me organized and to keep my credit rating good!

Grace Shaver
Bellaire, OH

Tip #5: Keeping up with bills—file in chronological order

I keep a box on my desk just big enough to hold my bills with one divider in it. In the front of the divider I keep the bills due, and behind the divider, I keep my checkbook, a few blank envelopes, stamps, address labels, and a pen. When the mail comes in, I immediately put the bills in the box. When I have time, I write the due date on the outside of the envelope and file them in chronological order. Every payday I take the bill from the front, pay it, and keep moving on to the next until all the bills due before next payday are paid. It might help to date the envelopes one week before the bill is due before filing them to make sure they get to their destination on time. This way you don't have to figure out post office travel time while paying them.

Jean Riskus
Green Bay, WI

Tip #6: Avoid late fees—stay focused

One thing I found I *had* to do was to separate my computer from my bill paying desk. I would start to pay bills and the computer would "call to me." Then, before I knew it, the bills were overdue, and I had spent all that time on the computer. Now the computer is in my kitchen. I can't be on it too long in there, and now my bills get paid as soon as they hit the mailbox. It's just easier for me that way.

Sandy
Attica, IN

Tip #7: Avoid late fees—use auto-pay

I would be in a terrible mess with bills and credit if it weren't for *auto-pay*. I have my checks directly deposited and my bills directly debited; I can't get late fees that way. So that the bills don't overdraw my account, I have those with set amounts come out of my checking account. Anything with a variable amount such as the phone bill gets charged automatically to my Visa. The utilities are on budget plans, so they are a set amount, and the credit cards each have a large enough set payment taken out each month to more than cover the minimum payment. Then when I get the credit card bill, I *do* pay additional amounts to reduce the balance or pay it off, but at least I *never* get charged a late fee.

Laura Tobin
Woodstock, IL

Saving Money

Tip #8: Balancing your checkbook—put money into a blind checking account

I used to have trouble balancing my checkbook and not knowing what the bank fees were (they fluctuated month to month). I had some checks bounce, so I decided to start blindly leaving money in the checking account. For example, if I made a check out for $14.45, then I would log in the checkbook that I actually wrote the check for $15. I did this for several months until I decided that I needed help, so I turned the checkbook over to a loan officer at the bank. The next day I went back to discover that over five or six months I had accumulated over $700 in the checking account! I thought this was a nice way to rehabilitate my problems with bounced checks and inadvertently save money at the same time.

NightStar
Kewanee, IL

Tip #9: Saving money—star special savings accounts
When saving for something big, start a Christmas club account. Most won't let you get to the money until a certain date, so you can save for a whole year! Use a payroll deduction or account debit when possible. That way you won't miss a payment!

Jamie Placito
Syracuse, NY

Tip #10: Balancing the checkbook—get an accountant
Many women (and men!) with AD/HD have a hard time balancing checkbooks, partly because the math gets in the way, but also because it's a detailed task and one that many procrastinate on. I often recommend that it's worth the money to find a bookkeeper to do this monthly; it's often less expensive than one thinks and has saved many a marriage.

Terry Matlen

Tip #11: Spending out of control—freeze your assets!
I am a shopping addict and have gotten into a lot of financial hot water over this. Now I keep my credit card in the freezer to prevent me from doing any impulsive shopping.

Koto Hayashi
Tokyo, Japan

Tip #12: Receipts—zip pouch

Purchase one of those vinyl school zippered pouches and keep it in your car to collect various receipts from stores, cleaners, etc.

Terry Matlen

Tip #13: Overspending on credit cards—change your habits

My credit cards are way over limit so I *had* to change my habits. First, I now force myself to only use cash. To pay off the cards, I took the one with the highest balance and paid an extra $25-50 per month on it until it was all paid off. Then I went to the next highest one and did the same. Only two more to go!

Karen Kruger
Chapel Hill, NC

Note from Terry

Money management problems are rampant in adults with AD/HD. Consider joining Debtors Anonymous. Details at: www.debtorsanonymous.org

---

Chapter 13

I've Just Seen a Face (But I Can't for the Life of Me Remember the Name): Memory Tips

No, you don't have Alzheimers, it just feels that way. Let's face it—memory issues come with the territory, but they don't have to paralyze you. Learn how others have managed.

Capturing Ideas

Tip #1: Reminders—post notes everywhere

> I put notes all over the place in areas where I see them that have to do with what I need to do. I wanted to put up corkboards more but still haven't done it. Tape works though. Use cork board squares to pin up reminders. They can go inside the kitchen cupboards if one does not want them showing.... but if they are cut in a diamond shape it looks cool on the outside, and they don't have to be big either.
>
> Tamarion

Tip #2: Record ideas—wall calendar

Post a calendar on the wall near your phone and use it to write appointments, household chores that have need to be done or *have* been done, birthdays, etc. Every time you answer the phone, you will see items you need to remember.

Tamara Gabrielsen
Halsey, OR

Tip #3: Remembering stuff—use your mobile phone

I tried to carry pencil and paper with me at all times in order to write down things that came to my mind before I forgot about them. Well, I never had that pencil when I needed it, but since I always carry my mobile telephone, I just put my "remembering-stuff" in the messenger outbox, and there it stays until I have carried out the actions. Sometimes help is closer than you think.

Siesta
Sweden

Tip #4: Memory—write on hand

You can make brief notes with a pen on your hand. This is especially good for short-term memory.

Tamara Gabrielsen
Halsey, OR

Tip #5: Remembering stuff—use a mantra

I use a mantra that I repeat over and over again: "What should I be doing now"?

Julia Greenbaum
Brooklyn, NY

Tip #6: Remembering appointments—put reminder in PDA day before

> When I put appointments in my Palm Pilot, I know that I can still forget to look at it! So I put a reminder on the previous day, "See tomorrow," especially if it's something unusual that I'm likely to miss.

Deborah Lancaster
Sunnyvale, CA

Tip #7: Remembering car maintenance—masking tape reminders

> To remember oil changes or tire rotations, use a piece of masking tape and write the mileage needed for the future action and tape it near the instrument panel in the car.

Tamara Gabrielsen
Halsey, OR

Keeping Track of Things

Tip #8: Losing things—just hold on!

> I realized that I was often losing things around the house, and after I started taking medication (read: was able to pay attention), I saw that it was often because I had put things down without realizing it. Usually, this was because when I needed that hand free, I just got rid of what was in my hand so I could move on (read: without a clue) to the next thing.

> Once I became aware of this, I began to hold on to things until I could put them where I could find them again (obvious places such as the kitchen counter where they wouldn't be lost forever). Try and become aware of putting things down so you

can eventually learn to pay attention to *where* they end up or put them where you'll find them again.

Deborah Lancaster
Sunnyvale, CA

Tip #9: Losing stuff—electronic finding device
I used to say "Boy, I wish I had a gadget like I do on my phone that locates it by beeping until you find it!" Then my boyfriend came across this and bought one: Sharper Image "Now You Can Find It! "Wireless RF Electronic Locator. It's been a lifesaver. Too bad it doesn't fit on my glasses, but I will keep looking for a gadget that finds those too!

Susan Nellans
Atlas, Michigan

Tip #10: Remembering things—wrap a strap!
Use a purse as a reminder: If I have to take something with me in the morning to work, I utilize my shoulder strap purse. I wrap the shoulder strap around the item so that when I grab my purse, it'll pull the items with it. If it's *under* my purse, I might pick up my purse and forget the item.

Lila Kadaj
Dearborn, MI

Physiology of Memory

Tip #11: Remembering things—move eyes upward
When you are trying to remember something, move your eyes upward. Often in stressful test-taking situations, students stare harder at the paper on their desk. Instead, look up, as this has been said to stimu-

late the memory part of the brain. If you think about it, when you are talking with someone and forget a word or phrase, you automatically look up as you try and remember it.

RM
Portland, OR

Miscellaneous Memory Tips

Tip #12: Forgetting lunch—put keys next to lunch in fridge

As a full-time professional and a mother of two teens, there are a lot of things to remember every morning. It seems like I always remember everyone else's things but not mine. In order to ease the stress and time crunch of my "getting ready for school/work" morning routine, I began packing my lunches the night before. The problem then became that almost every day I would end up at work, or at least in the car on my way to work, when I realized that my beautifully packed lunch was, once again, sitting in the refrigerator at home! I finally solved that my putting my car keys *in the refrigerator* each night, next to my lunch. It has been nearly ten years of doing this, but it has prevented me from ever leaving without my lunch. Of course, there have been some mornings when I frantically hunted for my car keys before realizing where they were... and low and behold, there was that lunch of mine too!

Anonymous
Bloomfield Hills, MI

Tip #13: Memory

I use the bags that are made out of netting for carrying books to the library. I like the net bags so I can easily see what is inside; this way I don't forget to return items.

June Michaels
San Francisco, CA

Tip #14: Remembering items

If I am supposed to bring something somewhere, I put it in my car *right away*. Even if I forget a week later that I was supposed to bring a tent back to the scout meeting, it's already in my car and is only as far away as the parking lot.

Laura Tobin
Woodstock, IL

Math

Tip #15: Calculating tips—handy tip card

Math isn't my strong point; I can barely remember my times tables. So when it comes to leaving tips, I'm often at a loss. I've been using a plastic Tip Card for **years**; it's as small as a credit card and fits right into your wallet. You can look up a 15 or 20% tip and know within seconds how much to leave. You can order them at www.puffins.com (search for "tip": they are called "Tip Table Cards").

Terry Matlen

Tip #16: Remembering multiplication tables—go with what you know

To remember multiplication tables, just use the ones

you remember. For example, if you can't remember what 9 x 9 equals, then think 3 x 9 = 27, and 27+27+27 = 81.

Tamara Gabrielsen
Halsey, OR

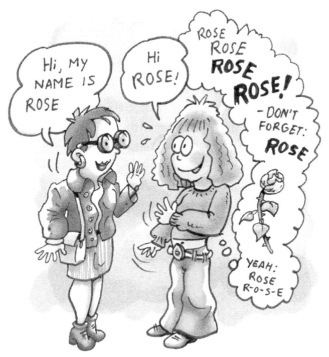

Names

Tip #17: Remembering names—repetition is key

When someone introduces me to a person, I can never remember the person's name. It's kind of like the old saying: "It goes in one ear and out the other." Now, I try and use their name three times in the conversation. For example, I might say, "Karen, I would like to introduce you to Brenda." "Nice to meet you,

Brenda. Are you from Louisville, Brenda? What kind of work do you do, Brenda?" Once I have said it three times, I have yet to forget. It works all the time.

Karen S. Fox
Louisville, KY

Tip #18: Remembering names—scroll down the alphabet
I can remember every birthday of every person I meet, but I have the hardest time with names. This is kind of a strange way to remember someone's name, but when I forget a name, I start going through the alphabet in my head, starting with "A." Most times when I reach the letter that the name begins with, it jogs my memory, and I come up with the correct name. It's not the most efficient way to remember a name...but then again...how often is an AD/HD brain ever "efficient!!!"

Heather
California

Tip #19: Remembering names—make a silly rhyme
Make a silly rhyme or associate a word with someone's name. For me, I remember the name Amanda by thinking Mandyroo (a warped kind of kangaroo).

Tamara Gabrielsen
Halsey, OR

Directions

Tip #20: Remembering directions—notebook in glovebox
Keep a small notebook in your glove compartment to jot down directions. That way you'll always know how

to get to where you have to go: doctors' offices, your child's friend's house, favorite shops, etc.

Trish Starsky
Holland, MI

Tip #21: Remembering locations—phonebook in car

Store an extra phone book in your trunk. I don't know how many times I've driven around in circles because I can't remember where the doctor's office, new restaurant, etc. are.

Candice Sholey
Topeka, KS

Tip #22: Remembering directions—make a file

Use the net and keep a file of directions to places you go out of town. You can even modify these directions using your word processing program and make a simple numbered list for each turn, etc.

Tamara Gabrielsen
Halsey, OR

Reminders

Tip #23: Mnemonics—Post-its

Let it be okay that some things are so important that they require Post-it notes absolutely everywhere, including the car steering wheel, the toilet seat, in the freezer—anywhere you think your eyes are going to see them. Also, putting a rubber band around my wrist helps me recall that I've got something to remember.

Donna Parten
Sacramento, CA

Tip #24: Remembering engagements—AOL Reminder Service

> In addition to making lists for everything, I have AOL and use the reminder service to make sure I remember to go to appointments, make phone calls, and remember important events.
>
> > Marie E Mendoza
> > Fall River, MA

Tip #25: Remembering needed items—two briefcases

> I use a two briefcase system: one for Monday, Wednesday, and Friday and one for Tuesday and Thursday. That way, I don't lose my books, and if I pick up the correct briefcase, I always have the necessary stuff with me.
>
> > Darla Wells
> > Lafayette, LA

Timers

Tip #26: Remembering things around the house —timer

> To prevent the kitchen from burning up when I forget to take things off the heat, I have a kitchen smoke alarm. I have posted a set of menus on my kitchen wall so I don't have to brainstorm about what to cook. I use the microwave timer for the laundry (time to add softener, time to get the clothes out of the washer and into the dryer, etc), as I live in an apartment and do not have my own washer and dryer.
>
> > Maykah Marshall

Tip #27: Remembering to give the animal meds—long-lasting injections

It's hard enough to remember to take my own medications let alone to give my animals their meds. So rather than forgetting to give my dogs their monthly heartworm preventative tablets, my veterinarian offered the option of giving a heartworm preventative via injection that lasts for six months called ProHeart-6. At the end of five months, they send me a reminder notice (or e-mail, or phone call) to bring the dogs in for another injection. No more worry that my dogs will get a fatal disease due to my forgetfulness!

Gudrun
Northern California

Chapter 14

Revolution: Technology

Technology: either you love it or you hate it. Personally, I love all the gadgets and electronics—they really can make life easier. But remember to only use what works for you! If you're a paper kind of gal, don't force yourself to use a Palm Pilot.

Creative Ways to Use a Palm Pilot

Periodically, I run a contest at my Web site (www.addconsults.com). Recently, I asked visitors to come up with creative ways to use their Palm Pilot and received quite a few innovative, unique responses. The first four tips below are the winners and honorable mentions from the contest, followed by regular tip submissions from other women.

First Place Winner: use it to lose weight
> I have used my Palm Pilot to help me lose 136 pounds in less than one year. How did I do that, you ask? I have software (by Healthetech) called BalanceLog (www.healthetech.com/balancelog/) that sets up a diet program for you based on your personal goals, metabolism, weight, age, etc. I track everything I eat

and all the exercise I do on there, and it holds me accountable so that I can lose weight. I don't leave the house without my Palm Pilot—after all, it has helped me cut my weight nearly in half in an amazingly quick and healthy way.

Autumn Conley

Second Place Winner: use it to have a baby!

The most unique thing I have used it for was to keep track of labor when I had my son, and I'll be using it for that again this summer! It's great. It sure has helped keep track of contractions, their length, and how frequent they were!!!!

Denise Layman

Honorable Mention #1: memory triggers for names

Meet with people repeatedly but infrequently? Consequently, you may have trouble remembering names. Palm Pilot can recap the location, people you're likely to encounter, their descriptive characteristics, and their names.

Ardith Mori

Honorable Mention #2: get that drat cat!

It works as a cat retardant since I can program it to do 'phaser fire' if the cat's on the computer again.

Kris Paige

Tip #1: Reminder of tasks—use the "endless repeat" function

I have entirely given up on using the "to do" list in my Palm Pilot because if I don't hit the "to do" button, I never see my list! Instead, I enter my things to do on my calendar (where I have to go every day of the work week, minimum!). I enter any given task with "no time" and put it on endless repeat (until I complete the task and get to delete it). That way I see my list every time I check my calendar, and I am reminded every day (great for when procrastination inevitably sets in!)

Laura
Scottsdale, Arizona

Tip #2: PDA—parking

I use a PDA to remember where I've parked.

Mary

Tip #3: PDA—various uses

I have to admit that I mostly use mine for the alarms. But I do keep my shopping list on it and can just delete items when I pick them up at the store. I also keep a list of authors that I like on it, so that when I get to the library or a bookstore, I can remember their names, especially if it is someone new to me. I keep my daughter's class list and parents' names in the address book. (I put the kids' names in an unused phone number slot, so that I can find the parent by the child's name.) And, finally, I play games on it when I am waiting around.

Corine
Ellicott City, MD

Tip #4: PDA—various uses

I use my Handspring for all of the following:
- Keeping track of cash spent instead of trying to hold onto all those receipts and little scraps of paper.

- Keeping a running list of questions I need to research and the answers I find for quick reference.
- Having a morning alarm clock with my intended "morning routine" to remind me of exactly why I decided it was necessary to get up so early!
- Brushing up on my Euchre skills for the next Midwestern competition.

Amanda

Tip #5: PDA—beepers

Mine has different beep tones so I use them as reminders for various things: one to remember to take my meds, one to pick up the kids, one to leave for work, etc.

Claudia Granowski
Marietta, GA

Tip #6: Reminders—various tips

Invest in a good PDA and carry it with you everywhere you go. All appointments can go in it with an alarm to go off in time for you to get ready and leave the house. It can be checked when making an appointment to make sure you're not over scheduling. If a thought comes to mind, put it in the memo section. If you see the medicine cabinets are getting dirty or the oven needs cleaning, put it in the to-do section. Shopping lists, wish lists, everything can go in this one little machine that you hold in your hand. I can't live without mine. If I didn't have a timer set for starting supper, my family would starve. No more need for notes all over the house. I used to spend more time writing out and organizing schedules and lists than actually doing the jobs. With a PDA, you can set it to repeat as often as you wish and forget about it until it reminds you.

Jean Riskus
Green Bay, WI

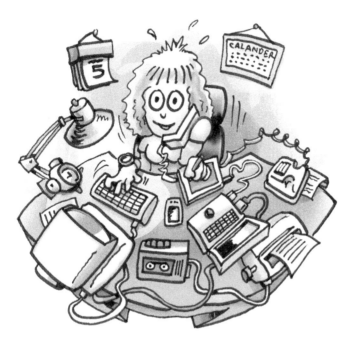

Internet, Computers, and Cell Phones

Tip #7: Storing files—Yahoo's additional storage option

I purchase additional storage on my Yahoo account for about $29 a year. This allows me to save and store my important files online. Instead of trying to keep up with paperwork, contact information, "how to" instructions, etc., I save it in my Yahoo briefcase, which is accessible from any computer. Also, most cell phones with online features can access Yahoo email. Paperwork still manages to pile up, but I can throw things away much easier knowing I have a copy stored online.

Kara C.

Tip #8: Remembering important dates—online reminder
Forget birthdays? Use an online birthday reminder service to help you remember (many are free). I use www.birthdayalarm.com, which reminds me via email of upcoming birthdays at intervals of one week and three days before each special day. The data input can be done manually or via the site's script (done automatically if you provide the email address). You have the flexibility to determine the frequency of notification and editing is a breeze. It has saved a few of my relationships! Within seconds of receiving the reminder, you can send off an email "Happy Birthday" to your special friend!

Joan Smith
Kalamazoo, MI

Tip #9: Forgetfulness—tie a "virtual" bow on your finger
On AOL 9.0, in the task bar at the top, is a 'remind me' icon with a fist, a raised finger and a bow tied around the finger. Set the timer to interrupt 'getting lost' online!

Irish Cookie
Long Island, NY

Tip #10: No time to shop?—shop online
Access information and shop online, for example, you

can buy movie tickets online rather than standing in line.

RM
Portland, OR

Tip #11: Reminders—MS Outlook Calendar's many uses

I use the Microsoft Outlook calendar reminders like a day planner or a Palm Pilot and put four reminders in it: one maybe on Friday, one the day before the appointment, one the day of the appointment early enough to see it in time, and one at the actual appointment time. With the copy and paste function, this can be done quickly. Also, you can use Microsoft Outlook's calendar program to enter library due dates and renew dates and then renew by telephone. It also pops up on my computer screen with constant naggers. If I don't delete them, it can be used like a to-do list and will pop up the next time you check your email. I get to delete them when I've accomplished my task.

Cathlin Darling-Owen
Dummerston, VT

Tip #12: Finding sale items—online deals

I rely on the computer for many things. I find great sales by going to various websites that compare prices for you (www.pricegrabber.com is one). When shopping online, you can also do a search for coupons by entering, for example, the words: "amazon coupon"). I've even found lost relatives online by searching my maiden name. And what would life be without eBay?

Terry Matlen

Tip #13: Airline travel—how to go online to get good seats

Since I have to travel a lot, I found a great trick for getting good airline seats. A day before I leave for my trip, I log online and check in for my flight. You usually can't do that until about 24 hours before the flight. Then (this is the good part), I check to see what seats are available and often am able to switch the seat I have to a much better one.

Peggy Horn
Brighton, IL

Tip #14: Reducing papers—use online manuals and scanning

Manuals for everything can now be found online. When I lose the manuals—which is nearly all the time—I go online rather than looking for it. This works for directions or rules to board games, too. And I scan everything—soccer team rosters, schedules, etc.—so when I need them, they are in the folder with my son's name on it and under "Soccer" with a folder titled with the team name and date. I've used it many times to look up phone numbers etc. I also scan the kids' artwork right away; then I can let it get lost in the house or wrecked. If they say something cute (the young ones, that is), it can go into the same type of folder.

Cathlin Darling-Owen
Dummerston, VT

Chapter 15

With a Little Help from My Friends: Humor for the Soul

If we take ourselves too seriously and see AD/HD as a crippling disease that leaves us incapable and broken, we will certainly fall into a self-fulfilling prophecy. Sometimes it helps to see the humor in situations, so when you're feeling particularly vulnerable or down, come back and reread this section.

You Know You Have AD/HD When...

You know you have AD/HD when...
> You are overjoyed that Blockbuster has done away with late fees so you can rent again.

> Teddy Benitez
> Bay Point CA

You know you have AD/HD when...
> You give directions to someone verbally, but they watch your hands to see which way you *really* meant for them to turn!

> Kris Paige
> Mosinee, WI

You know you have AD/HD when...

You are running late but really want coffee. You realize that you have no cash and have to go to the drive-through ATM machine. After being lucky enough to locate the card and get cash, you proceed to the coffee shop drive-through, which is a 90 second drive from the bank. After placing your order, you double check just to make sure you still have the money. It's a good thing you did because you can't locate the money.

You decide to be courteous and pull out of the line while you look for the money. After about two minutes you locate the money in a pocket of your wallet that you thought you looked through five times before. You then get back in the drive-through line and pull up to the window only to notice a very confused look on the coffee shop worker's face. After he asks you what your order was, you answer and begin apologizing for messing up the line.

Tara McGillicuddy
South Shore, MA

You know you have AD/HD when...

When I was in high school, I got dressed for school one morning and couldn't decide which shoes to wear with my outfit. So I tried one of each on and stood in front of the mirror trying to choose. I turned to the left, then the right, then straight ahead, over and over trying to make up my mind...then my mind went elsewhere, down some bunny trail until it was time for the bus. So out the door I ran, catching the bus right before it left my stop. As I walked down the aisle to a free seat, I was really pleased when one of the boys said "Hey, I like your shoes!" As I looked down to see which ones I had chosen, I was mortified to find that in reality I had forgotten to make any decision at all! I hurriedly got off the bus, walked home, put on matching shoes and walked my deflated ego to school.

I didn't think I would ever do that again, but I was wrong. I did it again in college. Even worse, when I was in the Navy, living off base, I drove to work, parked, and got ready to go inside...I had no shoes at all, only my stocking feet. Late as usual, I couldn't turn around and go home. I had no choice but to go in to my commanding officer in full uniform, except for no shoes and try to explain my predicament.

Fortunately, that was not the same week that I submitted a request chit for special liberty so that I could clean the bean sprouts from the beans that I had spilled several days earlier when I was cleaning and sorting beans for soup (this was the explanation I typed in the space for the reason). Now instead of beans in my sink, I had bean sprouts. My whole office was so amused that the request was approved, and I had the day to clean my kitchen.

Roberta Flood
Hobart, IN

You know you have AD/HD when...
On the way home from a restaurant my husband and I thought we had seen a man with a rifle walking around in a suburban area so we called the police department

to tell them what we saw. The police came and our house was *soooo* messy that they took one look at the apartment and thought we were either broken in to or that my husband and I had just had a terrible fight. The curtains were hanging half way off and there were jeans flung on top of the cabinets. They had come in a hurry because they had only received a 911 call and didn't know what they were there for. The police officer looked rather pissed off when he realized that this was how the house always looked and it wasn't as urgent as he thought.

Debbie Owens
Vermont

You know you have AD/HD when...

...you go to put on your winter coat at the *end* of your work day only to find a bra hanging off of the front of your coat, stuck to the Velcro. Oh, my gosh!!! Yes, I had walked into my school, (late) with a bra hanging off of my coat!!! All I can say is thank goodness I was late and a staff meeting was going on, otherwise many people would have seen my "interesting" addition to my coat! (*The down coat is off-white, and I'd just done the whites, pulled the coat out of the dryer, put it on, and raced off to work.) This is a true story!

Mary Kay L.
Batavia, IL

You know you have AD/HD when...

Every time you take a photo with your digital camera, it powers off; you then spend two days deciding whether you should buy new batteries or get the charger checked, only to find on day three that with each photo you take you are pressing the power button instead of the button to take the photo! You have owned this camera for two years and use it almost daily!!

Briana
Bristol, Qld. Australia

You know you have AD/HD when...

You are franticly looking in your purse for your cell phone and tell the person you are talking to on your cell phone what you are looking for!

When you go to the store to pick up your contact lenses. You spend an hour looking at everything in the store *including* the glasses frames and then leave. Halfway home you realize you forgot to pick up your contacts.

DeeAnna
Riverside, Ca

You know you have AD/HD when...
- You have committed to memory all the account numbers and expiration dates but forget to pay the bill.
- Your spouse lets you sleep late because they are tired.
- You can remember your friends phone number but not their last name.
- You can recite your driver's license number and/or social security a thousand times faster than remembering their last known location.

Tammy
Georgetown, TX

You know you have AD/HD when...

- You practice "intuitive checking:" if the car you're making payments on is still in your driveway, you still have time to write a check.
- You're so accident-prone that when friends can't get in touch with you by phone, they call the hospital.
- You are on a first-name basis with the locksmith.

Eve
San Marino, CA

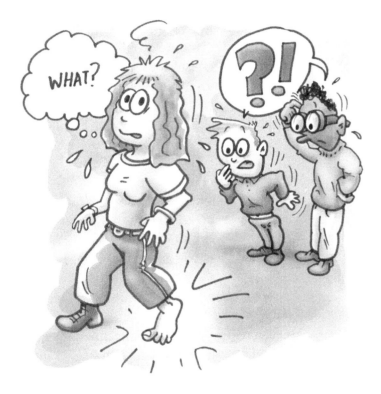

You know you have AD/HD when...

One time I decided to take my mother and kids on a day trip to Disney. As always I was working very hard at proving to my mother that I am a competent adult. All went well until we began unloading in the parking lot only to discover that I had no shoes. I searched feverishly throughout the car and trunk before confessing my foot problem. We loaded back in the car, drove to a tourist shop where I put on my mom's shoes and went in to purchased flip flops. A typical day in the life of ADD.

Carrie Houseman
Kissimmee, FL

You know you have AD/HD when...

You turned 24 on the 24th day of the month, and your two children share the same birthday as you and you have to ask them the day they are born. Short term memory issues—okay, sue me!!!

Frany Pelletier
Edmonton, Alberta
Canada

You know you have AD/HD when...

...you go to the grocery store for bread, and you come home with cereal, cheese, ice cream, paper towels, butter, apples, crackers, milk...and no bread. I'm sure many people have submitted this same example, but it happens to me *all* the time. I get *so* frustrated!

Heather
Laguna Niguel, CA

You know you have AD/HDwhen...

> I was looking through boxes of stuff in my garage for an upcoming garage sale when I discovered that I have three copies of the same book, *Attention Deficit Disorder in Adults* by Lynn Weiss!!! I have one hard copy and two soft cover copies. Guess I forgot that I had the book not once but twice. Imagine that. I am still laughing at myself over this.

Anonymous

You know you have AD/HDwhen...

> You have spent the last month planning your son's birthday day. You've had a busy day full of paperwork along with writing down dates, you fall into bed and then panic that your son's birthday is a day earlier than you thought because you can't remember the date! You need to get out of bed and go check the calendar. You get back to bed but can't remember what you just read on the calendar, so you send your husband to check so you can sleep at last.

Briana
Bristol, Qld. Australia

You know you have AD/HD when...

> ...you arrive at school (work) with *no shoes*. It was a warm spring day, and I'd had my sandals in my hand when I went out to the car. Before I got there, I remembered my lunch and ran back inside to grab some things out of the refrigerator. I put my sandals down to put these items into a bag, then ran out to the car and drove to work. I didn't realize until I arrived at work. So, I walked in barefoot. I asked various teachers and discovered one who happened to have an ex-

170

tra pair of sandals under her desk. But this was not until after my principal saw me in the hallway while she was talking to some parents!!! Arrrggghhh! I must say, I have since moved onto another job but that story still circulates there these many years later. Ah, well, such is life!

Mary Kay L.
Batavia, IL

You know you have AD/HD when...

After a marathon house cleaning day, you stop and realize that things are in worse disarray than before you began. All the chairs are pulled away from the table after vacuuming, piles of books are all around the bookcase from when you started to dust and sort, the stairs are heaped with things that belong upstairs but never made it back up there, the dining room table is sky high with things that have no real place to go because you stacked things there as you took them from the other rooms where they didn't belong. Your father, who often comes to help with home repairs, always brings his own tools because even though you have the same basic ones (tape measure, hammer, screwdriver, and such), he can never find anything he needs.

You know it is genetic when you have no trouble identifying your daughter's clothing at dance class because they are the only ones in the middle of the changing room floor.

Anonymous

You know you haveA D/HD when...

...the inside of the car windows are covered with dry-erase marker notes to yourself, and you tell your long-suffering spouse that it's cheaper than window tinting.

Kris Paige
Mosinee, WI

You know you have AD/HD when...

- You brush your teeth with Diaperene, that waxy stuff for baby bums.
- You put some music on the stereo and then walk out of the house and start gardening.
- You have to ask your kids, "Did you notice if I took my meds or not?"
- You finally remember to buy ketchup, and when you get home, you find you had already remembered to buy ketchup three times before.
- You can burn hard boiled eggs and don't remember even starting to cook them.
- You send your kids off to school and the neighbor calls out to tell you there is no school that day.
- You find yourself washing the cellar floor rather than writing that letter you have to do.
- You holler to the cat for doing something wrong but realize you just used your ADD son's name instead.
- You read at least three or four books at a time on different topics since meds have allowed you the ability to sit down and read for awhile.
- You explain that you are late for the appointment because you couldn't find your keys, but when

you reach in your waist pack to pay the bill, you suddenly see three sets of keys.

- You have trained your rain forest type plants to thrive in desert conditions.
- You don't lock your door for the obvious reasons that should anyone break in they will need good luck in finding anything or not tripping on the way out.

Anonymous

You know you have AD/HD when...

When I was in college I was really tired from staying up late when the studying had gotten really intense. I lived in apartments on campus where you could drive to classes or take the bus. When I woke up the next day to go to school, I went outside and looked for my car. It wasn't there. I said, "Holy sh*t, MY CAR WAS STOLEN." It took me at least five minutes to realize that I had forgotten and taken the bus home from classes and didn't even think once about where my car had spent the night.

Debbie Owens
Vermont

You know you have AD/HD when...

You ask a stranger, "Can *you* read what I wrote?" while pointing to your grocery list.

Hi NRG
Virginia Beach, VA

You know you have AD/HD when...

You've "lost" your watch—again!—and your eight year old says," Mom, think in your head where was the last time you put it." I found it two weeks later in the bathroom closet without a clue how on earth as to how it got there!!

Bette K.

You know you have AD/HD when...

If you could remember to pick up your prescription for Ritalin, you could remember to pick up your prescription for Ritalin.

Jan DeLaura
Norfolk, VA

You know you have AD/HD when...

You put your children in time out for two minutes and when they are done, *you* forgot why they were there in the first place.

Anonymous

You know you have AD/HD when...

I went thru the toll booth and sat and waited for the toll operator to hand me the ticket. I waited, and he waited. Finally, he said, "You have to hand me the ticket." I was supposed to pay him!

Debbie Owens
Vermont

You know you have AD/HD when...

- It actually cost less to purchase a book than to check it out at the library and pay the inevitable late fees.
- The most important question to ask when interviewing a new doctor or dentist is: "Do you

call your patients the day before to remind them of the appointment?"

Anonymous

You know you have AD/HD when...

You're the navigator but despite past performances you get totally lost only to find out that you landed at *the other airport* in town and are now about 50 miles out of your way. The standard joke quickly becomes "You mean the *other* airport?" even if there's only one.....

Kris Paige
Mosinee, WI

You know you have AD/HD when...

You get up to do or get something and by the time you get to the other room you have forgotten what you meant to do and you have to go back to where you were and sit in the same spot to figure it out.

Jan DeLaura
Norfolk, VA

You know you have AD/HD when...

You lock your keys in you car, call *AAA*, and forget what town you are in.

Tara McGillicuddy
South Shore, MA

You know you have AD/HD when...

You're walking through the grocery store with your kids, and someone passing by says "Hi," so with great enthusiasm and a big smile you reply, "Hi, how are you?" A moment later your kids ask, "Mom, who was that?" and you reply, "I have no clue!"

Anonymous

You know you have AD/HD when...

You call someone and get their answering machine and half-way through leaving your phone number all of a sudden it doesn't sound right, so you stop and then blank out completely and can't *remember* your phone number. So you hem and haw a bit, then tell the person you were calling that they will have to look it up in the phone book.

Corine
Ellicott City, MD

You know you have AD/HD when...

You are searching all through the refrigerator for the spaghetti sauce you *know* you just bought and could not possibly have used up already, finally slam the fridge door in bewilderment, and see the jar sitting on the counter six inches away from you where you obviously just put it (it's still cold), but you don't remember even seeing it before. Aaarrrgggh!

Anonymous

Stories to Tickle the Funny Bone

Your mother's favorite story to tell is when you were about four years old sitting in the seat of the grocery shopping cart while shopping with her. When checking-out, the clerk said, "Hi, little girl. What's your name?" and you replied, "Elizabeth-don't-do-that."

Duckling

Joke: Two ADDers were sitting at the table of the local diner and their conversation drifted from politics to cooking. "I got a cookbook once," said one, "but I could never do anything with it." "Too much fancy work in it, eh?" asked the other. "You said it. Every one of the recipes began the same way: 'Take a clean dish...'"

Anonymous

I can't believe what I just did. I went to weigh myself, stood on a stool, and looked down at my feet to see the numbers. OOPS—smack me in the head! Duh.

Jen
Minneapolis, MN

Life is too short to stuff a mushroom

Storm Jameson

When my car was broken into, the crooks only took a Walkman out of the back seat, but they emptied the glove box, apparently looking for whatever they could steal. My car was normally in such a state of dishevelment—papers strewn on the passenger seat and floor—that I didn't even know it had been broken into until I looked in the glove box for something!

Donna R.N.
Encinitas, CA

I have several places with keys placed around the yard for when I forget where the first hidden key is.

Debbie Owens
Vermont

I was proud of myself. I'm up, I'm dressed, hair is done and I'm going Christmas shopping for the family at the mall. Three hours later, I get back in the car and see my list on the passenger seat. I shopped, and I didn't get one gift. But I now have a new sweater and fleece jacket. Talk about stress. Christmas is Thursday. This is Wednesday. Merry Christmas!?

Blanche Rogers
Danbury, CT

Kitchen Chaos

Below are some delightful stories gathered from clients, friends, and acquaintances by my colleague in the field of AD/HD, author Kate Kelly, and myself. Enjoy them and hope they never happen to you!

In the last week, I opened the freezer door to find one shoe that I purposely put in to freeze a price sticker on the bottom of it in order to remove it. Five minutes time was my intention and a sufficient amount of time to accomplish my sticker removal technique. Needless to say, I had forgotten about it for days, as well as the fact that I had a new pair of shoes waiting to be worn. I also found a hand held mirror in the freezer that is normally stored in the bathroom closet. Why I put it in there, I still don't know!

Amy Pappalardo
Farmington, CT

Have you ever seen a blue chicken? I took a chicken out of the freezer one day, but I had cats, so I put the chicken in the oven (!) to defrost. I didn't turn it on or anything, just kept it from the cats. And from sight.

For a week. In July. Let me tell you, thank goodness for tight sealing freezer bags...but do you know how far they'll blow up before they actually explode? All of a sudden I remembered it, opened the oven door and almost puked. The bag was all puffed up, and the chicken was blue and green. I put it in a pail (didn't break the seal) and brought it down to the woods behind the garage....far behind!

Rexanne B. Mehler

I remember being in my first apartment and finally free of any parental authority. Unfortunately, during my years at home the kitchen was the last place I wanted to be. Well, I went to wash my first load of dishes and saw that I didn't have any dishwashing detergent, but aha!, I had Palmolive. Okay, great, now I can wash dishes, so I put a full amount of Palmolive in the little receiving chamber (ever heard of "A little dab will do ya?"—well, it's true). Anyway, I started the load and went to watch my favorite TV shows. I got a phone call a few minutes later and went to the kitchen to get it. Guess what! I had a thick layer of the sudsy stuff all over my little kitchen. I started laughing hysterically! The guy on the other end of the phone never called me back after that. I guess he realized I wasn't Suzie Q Homemaker! I have never seen a floor shine that much in my life!

Becky

About six years ago, I made tuna helper for supper one night when it was just my daughter and myself home. We ate it and had no problems. We thought that it tasted kind of different but couldn't pin-point just *what* it was ... *until* later on we were in the kitchen and found the can of tuna sitting there on the counter. To this day, we still kid about our having "helper" for supper.

D. Jennelle Kristyak

When I was first married in 1990, I was already in a panic about the post-honeymoon crash coming after only one month of marriage. I scrambled to use my creativity to keep the marriage "alive and interesting." I had decided to make an interesting meal that my husband would not soon forget! I decided to make cookie cutter meatloaf men decorated with vegetables for anatomically correct body parts. Imagine two peas here and a green bean there...need I explain further? I cut and shaped my meatloaf men and laid my soldiers in perfect form onto a cookie sheet. With my inexperience in the kitchen and my lack of motivation to seek help from a cookbook, it was inevitable that it would be a disaster. My meatloaf soldiers came out of the 450 degree smoking oven looking like corpses from a nuclear attack. The entire platoon was burned to a crisp on the outside and steak tartar on the inside.

Amy Pappalardo
Farmington, CT

10 Things to Never Do in the Kitchen (with no apologies to David Letterman)

10. Never get the ice cream out of the freezer while thinking of something else. By the time you remember it, not even the cat will drink it.

9. Never buy any cooking utensil that might be

harmed by scorching—especially Teflon coated ones that smell terrible when forgotten.

8. Never have just *one* timer set for a cooking project—set one in the kitchen and clip the other to your belt and set them both to the same time. This way you stand half a chance of getting back in the kitchen before whatever it was turns to charcoal.

7. Never use the same pan that you tie-dyed your daughter's t-shirt in to cook the mashed potatoes. Purple potatoes are not a gourmet food item.

6. Never cook without a large box of baking soda close by—this will put out most cooking fires without blowing up the house. Do not listen to your mother, who tells you to use flour (this *will* explode).

5. Never substitute ingredients, especially if company is coming. Using Ex-lax for the chocolate mousse is especially bad. Three trips to the store may save your marriage, your husband's job, and the visit from the rescue squad.

4. Never leave the house if you've been in the kitchen in the last hour. This lessens the chances of a phone call that starts with, "Honey, could we spend the next week in a motel while the insurance company rebuilds the house??"

3. When following a new recipe, if it says "preparation time two hours," find another recipe or get it at the store. There's no way that your concentration will last that long!

2. Never read Martha Stewart—she can't possibly be ADD or even real. She's a marketing image

created by Stephen King.
Drumroll, please!
The number one thing to never do:
1. Never, ever buy a house with a "gourmet
   kitchen" the size of a travel trailer. For one
   thing, you'll never find your way out (been
   there, done that). You'll also spend far too
   much time trying to figure out where you put
   the oregano. Far better to marry a man who
   cooks (Paul Prudhomme, maybe??) or find a
   nice little store that makes meals and delivers!

Kris Paige
Mosinee, WI

One evening I decided to make my fiancé a wonderful candlelight dinner with several courses. He had just gotten home from a long day at work and was sitting on the couch watching TV. To start the rice, I put water on to boil and then pre-heated the oven. Once that was finished, I began to give the dining room a more romantic atmosphere. I suddenly noticed an awful smell; it was like metal mini blinds burning on the heater (that my friends, is a different story). I ran to the kitchen. It was filled with thick black smoke. I ran to the stove to see how I had managed to burn rice in such a creative way. When I reached the stove, I suddenly noticed that I had forgotten to take the burner cover off. Of course, as I was waving away smoke with one hand and removing the charred burner cover with the other one, my fiancé walked in and said, "Wow, honey, dinner smells better than usual!" What a sweet guy!

Megan
Wenatchee, WA

I should know better than to put something on the stove to cook and walk away from it, thinking, of course, "Oh, I'll remember it!" *Sure, I will*! I put eggs and potatoes on to boil for potato salad and walked into the bedroom to clean it. Sometime later I heard a loud noise and couldn't figure out what it was. *Still* forgetting I had something on the stove, I walked out to the kitchen and WHOA! The water in the pan of potatoes had completely boiled away, and the bottom of the pan was totally burned. But the worst part? The noise I had heard was the eggs exploding! All over my stove, the refrigerator next to it, the wall, the floor. What a mess! And the smell? ARRRRRRGH! Oh, and we didn't have potato salad for dinner, either!

Pat Hall

Quotes from the Impatient Patients

Many thanks to my professional colleagues who have saved these interesting, funny, and often thought-provoking quotes from their patients.

Doc, what's the name of that memory drug you put me on?
Doctor: "Are you indecisive?"
Patient, turning to husband: "I'm not indecisive, am I?"

When a mom is asked how she knows her 20-old college student is inattentive, she answers, "She stops at *green* lights."

She has a piling system, not a filing system.
Husband of an AD/HD woman

My brain is like a washing machine stuck on the spin cycle.
Woman with AD/HD

I see the forest. I just keep bumping into the trees.
Physician with AD/HD

I talk so fast sometimes I say things I haven't thought of yet.
Businesswoman

My son's more AD/HD than I am. I'm a human being; he's a human *doing*.
40-year-old RN

I get to the end of paragraphs more.
Newly treated AD/HD college student

When I zone out, my brain goes to ADDland, and my body goes to the refrigerator.
College professor

Doctor: "Did you declare a major while in college?"
Patient: "Sure, lot's of them."
22-year-old college sophomore
after four years of college

It's like carrying around a 24-hour party in my brain!
Patient with Bipolar, AD/HD, Tourette, OCD

It's like there's no background noise; it's *all* fore-ground noise.

28-year-old mother

If *I'm* controlling it, it's white noise. If I'm not, it's just noise, and it doesn't matter *how* other people clas-sify it.

Anonymous

I even lose interest in the stuff I'm interested in.

24-year-old college student

You mean I'm 'sposed to *think about* stuff before I *do* it??????

Anonymous

When asked why she talks so much out of turn, a young student answered, "I need something for my mouth to do."

I thought the other people were the problem—they talk about one thing too long! I'm always afraid that the subject of the conversation is going to change be-cause in my mind it's about to.

Newly diagnosed artist and mother

I've got piles and piles of piles in piles.

Businesswoman

It's like over-dreaming; my dreams are so strong they wake me up.

Special Education Teacher

I major in minor things.

Forester

If you don't live on the edge, you can't see the view.

High-school senior

We're the "Uh-oh!" family.

Housewife and mother

Regarding coordination: "I trip over lint."

Security system worker

I have brain jumps.

Female patient

I figured she'd have nothing left but stumps for legs by the time she got out of there, the way she was kicking around inside me.

Mother of 15-year-old AD/HD girl,
when discussing her pregnancy

If I just had a speedometer on my thoughts…!

Anonymous

My mind is all dressed up with no place to go.

AD/HD Mother

My mind isn't racing at bedtime, but it sure is jogging!

Schoolteacher

The Atlanta airport? That's my house!

Anonymous

Trying to hold him as a child was like trying to cuddle a four-wheel-drive truck.

Mother of AD/HD child

I have moments of clarity in my world of obscurity.

38-year-old woman

He hardly eats, but it's not his appetite; it's his activity. At the table, his forks dance and his chicken fingers talk to one another.

Mom of 5-year-old with
untreated AD/HD

Doctor: Why do you think you eat more when you're bored?
Patient: It keeps my mouth busy.

Nursing student

The slide show is gone.

X-ray tech who before medication
could not get to sleep at night
due to running brain

AD/HD Definition of Hell: When you can't be *doing* anything!

Undiagnosed AD/HD Adult

I have the want-to; I just don't have the stick-to.

35-year-old AD/HD patient

Sometimes my brain feels like a superball in a racquetball court!

40-year-old professor

Whichever way he looks is the way he goes. You should see him when he's driving a boat!

Wife of an AD/HD artist

I live in sticky note hell!

Manager

I get bored of things I'm interested in!

24-year-old exotic dancer

Now I don't feel like I'm twenty feet behind the back of the room.

20-year-old college student

I still have all my piles, but I can *find* stuff in the ones I've made since I've been on the Concerta.

Physician

Doctor: Are you much of a packrat?
Patient: I save dust.

36-year-old housekeeper and mother

I'm always afraid that the subject is going to change because in my mind it's about to.

47-year-old artist and mother

I thought the *other* people were the problem—they talk about one thing for too long!

AD/HD mom

Most *unexpected* answer yet to the following question:

Doctor: So what's the best thing about being on Adderall after your first month?

Patient: My foot isn't sore every night.

> 40-year-old schoolteacher
> who stopped jiggling her foot
> for the first time in her life

Can't somebody stop the little drummer?

> Bipolar patient with untreated AD/HD

I *do* wish my brain would quit taking vacations without me!

> Adult with AD/HD

I stop to think, and then I forget to start again.

> Bumper sticker

I call him my ping-pong machine.

> Mother of three-year-old who had been
> asked to leave four daycare centers,
> describing how he bounces off the walls

Pardon me, doc; I was just doing a little brainsurfing.

> AD/HD teenager

When the medicine runs out, it's like somebody throws a sheet over my brain.

> Anonymous

I think I know what I want to do, and then the committee in my head starts talking.

> Dental assistant

She played in eggs a lot.

> Mom of very hyperactive 5-year-old,
> when asked to characterize her
> daughter's earlier years

I don't wear clothes; they wear me.

> Woman with tactile hypersensitivity

I'm distractible as h_ _l! Lock me in a black sound-proof room with no lights and only a computer to work with and I'd be counting the pockets in the egg crate insulation or the pixels on the screen!

> AD/HD bipolar engineer

She loves to entertain those nearby.

> A mom's graceful way of describing
> her inattentive-AD/HD 12-year-old's
> penchant for talking too much

I keep a lot of planes in the air; I just don't land any of them!

> AD/HD Bipolar Engineer

I got a call yesterday afternoon from the school nurse. My son was in her office complaining of a stomach ache. When asked why he was feeling sick, he indicated that "It might be the glue." Apparently, his class had a special presenter in their room yesterday morning and in an attempt to remain quiet for the presentation, he glued his lips shut.

> Mother of AD/HD child

Her first-grade teacher called her "Spring-Bottom."
> Mother of second grader who fulfilled
> criteria for out-of-seat behavior

It's like having mental ankle weights!
> 36-year-old woman, speaking of mild
> persistent depression (dysthymia) from AD/HD

There are days when I work and days when I try to work.
> College professor describing her
> professional work before Adderall

Chapter 16

Help:
Tips from Coaches and Professional Organizers

Experts agree that the optimal treatment for adult AD/HD is a combination of therapy, medication (if needed), psychoeducation, and support. Support often includes the help of an AD/HD coach and/or a professional organizer. Coaches, in particular, can be immensely helpful in showing you how to not get in your own way, how to prioritize and manage projects, and how to hold yourself accountable by keeping regular phone/email contact with them. It's not therapy but rather a pragmatic way to get through your day with a game plan. In this chapter, I asked some top coaches and professional organizers to share tips they use with their clients who have AD/HD.

Tips from Professional Coaches
Linda S. Anderson, M.A., MCC
Business and Personal Coach/Getting Clear
Specializing in Coaching AD/HD Professionals

Vice President, Attention Deficit Disorder Association
Doylestown, PA
Linda@gettingclear.com
www.gettingclear.com

Tip: Break any task down into five easy pieces.

Making changes or transitioning into an undesirable task like picking up all those papers can be excruciatingly painful to contemplate, let alone begin. The mind balks, "Where do I start?" It ruminates, "I can't. I can't." Finally, it runs away screaming, "It's hopeless!" So, try this. I call it five easy pieces. It has become a time-honored and much revered tool in my toolbox. Tell yourself when staring at that pile of paper, "I'll just do five easy pieces." Start with the really easy ones such as an envelope that gets thrown out, a bill that gets put with the other bills, a coupon with the coupons, etc. Start easy, aim for just five, and then pat yourself on the back. You can use five easy pieces just before a phone call, right after lunch, or first thing in the morning. Make it is easy and walk away with a completion, which is so much better than living with "I can't" and "It's hopeless." It's just five easy pieces.

Tip: Use affirmations to get clear.

These are affirmations for individuals who are truly challenged by the thought, let alone the task, of letting stuff go and of changing old patterns. You can choose the affirmations from this list that mean the most to you or design your own around any part of your life that you wish to change. State what you want to have happen in the positive, as if it is already happening. No one can stop you from pretending as if the things you wanted to have happening are happening right at that moment and that you are feeling great about it. Tape them, listen to them, or say them out loud while looking in a mirror. Let them reach into those inner areas of the brain that begin to reconnect the little dendrites in healthy supportive ways and celebrate yourself because you matter! (See Appendix for list of affirmations.)

David Giwerc, MCC, ICF

President of ADDA (Attention Deficit Disorder Association, www.add.org).
Master Certified Coach and the Founder/ President of ADDCA (ADD Coach Academy, www.addca.com)
Slingerlands, NY

Tip: Use music to ignite and rev up your engine.

Try using music to make boring tasks pleasant. The music's melodies and rhythms can create a second wind of energy that can empower you to do all kinds of things you might have otherwise put off. Why not target specific types of music for select tasks? Try using classical music for writing articles or reading since it doesn't have lyrics; many clients tell me that they cannot listen to lyrics when they are writing or reading as they are too distracting. Some people use jazz for brainstorming new concepts or use Motown or rock to exercise or do the dishes.

Tip: Develop your ability to focus by exploring your passions.

Find your area of passion or interest and observe how you are able to pay attention in those situations. Break down the steps that are essential to improving your ability to concentrate by asking the following questions:

- What subjects, topics, or tasks are you able to focus on?
- What steps are necessary for you to comprehend the object of your focus?
- What steps are necessary for you to complete the task of your focus?
- Do you tend to hyper focus on these types of tasks?
- Do these types of situations or tasks make it difficult for you to transition "out of" what you are focusing on and "into" what ever it is you need to be doing?

Now write them down in a format that works for you, e.g., visual map or recording it. By identifying and focusing on specific situations of interest, you stimulate you brain and gain the necessary internal momentum that will motivate you to complete a variety of tasks.

Tip: Take 24.

Take 24 hours to make a decision on important matters. There are very few situations that require anyone to make a decision on the spot. Because of your impulsive nature as an individual with ADD, it is important for you to pause and ask the question, "How will my answer or response to the request to serve my best interests?" Give yourself permission to "respond" rather than "react."

Tip: Discover and learn to use your natural learning styles.

Find a well- trained coach to help you identify your

learning/processing style, the way you take in and understand information and stimuli, and how you learn. There are six modes of processing or learning styles: visual, verbal, kinesthetic, conceptual, auditory, and tactile. For example, in college I would sing (verbal, auditory, dominant style) my class notes while rocking in my rocking chair (kinesthetic, preferred style), which helped me sustain focus on my notes. Ask yourself the following questions:

- What do I have to do in order to pay attention?
- What topics naturally sustain my attention?

When you identify the areas that you can pay attention in, you can learn the process that you use and apply it to other areas of your life. Follow up questions might include the following:

- What happens when I am able to focus on these topics or areas of interest?
- Do I need to move around in order to pay attention?
- Do I need music?
- Do I need to draw a picture or squeeze something?
- Do I need to read it out loud and have some one mirror or repeat it back in their words?
- What do I have to do in order to understand what I am paying attention to?
- Do I need to have questions answered first before I can go on to the next stage?

Tip: Reframing Ineffective Thinking with ADDentifiers
Definition
ADDentifiers are words that seem similar in meaning

but when articulated identify the shifts the ADDer is missing. ADDentifiers describe the lower level of functioning and encourages one to move up to the next level.

Perfection vs. Excellence
Perfection is about prejudging the outcome before you even start the task or goal. It is focusing on doing things so perfectly that you never get anything done. Perfection does not exist. It is an unrealistic expectation that cannot be achieved. Excellence is a realistic achievable standard that can be completed within a realistic timeframe.

Doing Things Right vs. Getting Things Done
Doing things right is a behavior that promotes procrastination, i.e., "If I can't do it perfectly or be the best at what I am going to do, I won't do it at all." This type of internalizing impedes any type of progress or action. When you complete projects or accomplish goals and tasks without worrying about the consequences or doing it perfectly (black or white thinking), you are getting things done. By completing tasks, you feel satisfied and learn from the momentum you have created. .Don't worry about doing things right; just get things done!! You'll feel better.

Can't vs. Won't
Can't really means you can't do something in the way a person who has Polio can't walk or a person who is blind can't see. *Can't* is a physical or neurological handicap. *Won't,* however, is a reaction, based on an inherently learned ADD weakness (black and white

thinking, procrastination, or poor self-esteem). *Won't* is the defeatist attitude that you are incapable of accomplishing a specific task or activity. *Won't* means you can be convinced with effort (proper systems, language, distinctions, advising challenging, listening, success stories, or identifying) to giving it a try.

Finish vs. Complete

Finishing a task is your perception of having completed the project. In reality, there may still be elements left undone for someone else to complete. When you complete a project, task, or goal, it is done in its entirety and you will not have to go back to finish the job or even think about it.

Gulp vs. Sip

For entrepreneurs, gulping is a dangerous way to run a business. If the business were a glass of water, the entrepreneur's enthusiasm and impulsivity would *gulp* all the water immediately. Once that water had been gulped, the business would have depleted its entire reserve. It is better for the entrepreneur to *sip*, savoring each experience, monitoring and protecting his or her reserve, and developing a rational plan rather than following an impulsive reaction.

Mary Jane Johnson, PCC
Professional Certified Coach
Toledo, OH
mjjaddcoach@Yahoo.com
www.addcoaching.com

Tip: Use a daily review checklist.

To make sure that clients are focused and on task throughout the day, I have them look at what is in front of them and ask themselves the following questions:

1. Is this important right now?
2. When does this need to be completed?
3. Am I making the best use of my time?
4. What else do I need to be doing?
5. Do I need to take a five minute break?
6. Should I continue with this task?
7. Do I need to be somewhere else right now?
8. What can I accomplish or wrap up in the time I have left?

It is helpful for them to use a timer set for every hour (or every half hour if needed) throughout the day so that they are reminded to use the checklist periodically. I have made these checklists up for clients (about the size of a 3" x 5" index card) and had them laminated. I suggest that they put them up in several places as a reminder to review their checklist.

Tip: Make a mini-agenda for phone calls.

For those of us with ADD, whether at home or at work, making just one phone call can easily use up an hour of our time. Between lack of focus and free flight of ideas, we can be all over the place. Often by the time we end the call, we may not have even touched on the subject or question we were calling about. To help stay focused and on task when making or returning phone calls, try using a mini-agenda for each call. Plan ahead for what you are going to say and the amount of time you will spend on each call. Set a timer or vibrating watch for that amount of time before you make the call. To make up mini-agendas for my clients, I take a piece of 8 _" x 11" paper and divide it into four squares with the following info: (See below)

Mini-agenda for Phone Calls

Date: _____ Time of call:_____

Person being called:_____

Phone number:_____

Points to cover (1, 2, 3):

_____

_____

_____

Response or action (1, 2, 3):

_____

_____

_____

Limit of minutes (circle): 5, 10, or 15

Outcome: Left message ____ or _____

Call back _____ Date _____ Time_____

I also tell them to take a few minutes to transfer the response/action of each call to his or her calendar, to do list, or wherever it needs to go once all calls are made. If they need to keep records of certain phone calls, they can cut them from the sheet and place them in the appropriate file (or make up each mini-agenda on a single sheet for easier filing).

Jennifer Koretsky
New York, NY
jennifer@addmanagement.com
www.ADDmanagement.com

Tip: Avoid absolutes, negative thoughts, and rumination.

Have you ever told a partner, "You're always late!" or complained to a friend "You never call me!?" Thinking and speaking in absolutes like "always" and "never" makes the situation seem worse than it is and programs your brain into believing that certain people are incapable of delivering. Also in keeping with dealing with negative thoughts is the idea that your thoughts can't hold any power over you if you don't judge them. If you notice yourself having a negative thought, detach from it, witness it, and don't follow it. Along the same lines, if you find yourself ruminating, a great way to stop it is to interrupt the pattern and force yourself to do something completely different. Rumination is like hyper-focusing on something negative. It's never productive because it's not rational or solution-oriented, it's just excessive worry. Try changing your physical environment; go for a walk or sit outside. You could also call a friend, pick up a book, or turn on some music.

Tip: Plan the time to tackle a chore.

When you plan to tackle a task, break it down into simple steps that make it less overwhelming. Here's an example I like to use: cleaning a cluttered and disorganized closet. Before you ever open the closet door, set aside 15 minutes that you can use to write down some steps such as the following:

1. Donate or throw out all clothes that I haven't worn in the past year.
2. Designate the right side of the closet for work clothes and the left side for casual clothes.
3. Hang belts, scarves, and other accessory items in the middle of the closet.
4. Arrange shoes neatly on the closet floor.
5. Remove all non-clothing items from the closet.

Taking the time to break down the task into 3 or more steps makes the act of cleaning out a closest nothing more than a simple system to follow. It relieves pressure and often prevents that feeling of being overwhelmed by the mess.

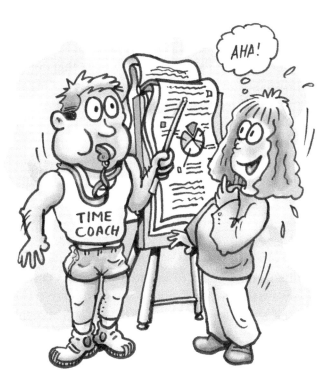

Kerch McConlogue, CPCC
Board member for ADDA (Attention Deficit Disorder
Association)
Baltimore, MD
kerch@mapthefuture.com
www.mapthefuture.com

Tip: Use the task and notes tools on your PDA.
If I come across a book I want to read, I can look it up
in our library's online database. I copy out the title,
author, and call number and store it as a task with a
library category. Then when I go to the library, I remember what I want to look for and where to find it.
(This also helps me not to go directly to Amazon and
buy the book!) I also include directions to meetings
in the notes section of the record. But there is a big
problem with actually being able to read that little
print, so more than likely I will print that out. Sometimes, however, I would like to test its ability to skim
the water like a flat rock! I don't care if it floats!

Tip: Make up a master list for traveling.
Make a list of every single thing you have to take
with you on repeatable trips. Pack the list with a major thing you always need and check it before you
leave. If it's camping, put the list with the tent.

On a recent trip to a car show, my client (OK, really
this is me) packed food and drinks in a cooler which
always traveled in the back seat of the convertible and
used a plastic container full of ice for a coolant. But
no matter what they say, plastic ware leaks. And it

made a mess. DUH! Freezer blocks are a *much* better choice, but they weren't on the list of things to take, so she filled the plastic ware.. and YUK!

She says, "I'll have to put that on the master list." He says, "Why? That should be a no brainer!" She says, "Ideas pour through my brain just like melted ice in the cooler! I'll write it down."

Tip: Keep a travel bag of toiletries packed and ready to go.
My father had a shaving kit with travel sizes of all his normal supplies. He had nothing to add; he just grabbed the kit when he packed for a trip. I don't have the luxury of two sets of make up, but the other stuff is always together in a clear makeup bag. It makes it a lot easier to pack.

Tip: Visualize your whole day.
When planning a busy day, or even a not so busy one, list the errand/tasks to be done *today only*. Think about where you have to be to do each one, what you have to have, and especially how long each task will take. Then put the pieces together like a puzzle. In what order will you go to the bank, the cleaners, and the grocery store? Are there any tasks that are constrained by the time of day? Do the cleaners close early on Tuesday? If you have to wait at the pharmacy, can you read an article you were meaning to get to? Once you have mapped the day, it's much easier to keep on task because then it's just a matter of getting started— and not so much of a problem to finish.

Tip: Use a white board to sketch out menu, ingredients, and timing of a meal.

I make a list on the big white board in my kitchen of all the food I'll be serving at a big meal. I can think it all out clearly and see it all there. It always amazes me how *few* items are really on that list. Then I back plan when each thing should go in the oven for how long and whether or not it can be warmed up. The list is a reminder when me—or my helpers—are actually carrying food to the table. Plus it lets other people help me remember all the parts.

Kris Paige
Mosinee, WI
kris@addragonflycoaching.com
www.addragonflycoaching.com

Tip: Use a timer to help you manage chores.

Grab your timer and time how long it takes to get done with something you hate to do—like cleaning the bathroom. It probably takes less time than you thought. Then, when that chore needs to be done, set the timer and tear through it. Bingo! Double reward: it's done, and it hasn't eaten up the whole day!

Tip: How to prepare and use a list for grocery shopping.

Print a list of what you always use such as brands of cereal, milk, bread, eggs, cuts of meat, veggies, etc. Post this on the inside of the cabinet next to the refrigerator or inside the pantry door. Check off when you run low. Grab the list and head to the store. If you put the list in a sheet protector and use a dry erase marker, it becomes an easy way to keep the cupboard full!

Tip: Write reminders on your car window in dry erase marker.

Really need to remember something in the morning or after work? Use a dry-erase marker to write it on your bathroom mirror or the *side* window of your car! Write it where you'll look, (don't write anything personal on the window like "Pick up money from acct #......"), then erase with a quick swipe of a tissue when it's done. You can use different colors for different chores or different colors for different folks. You can also leave quick, thoughtful messages for others in your family this way!

Tip PDA—various uses.

- Record catalog numbers of possible gift ideas from catalogs you don't get.
- Beam your business card to others.
- Quickly note directions before you get lost for the third or twenty-third time.
- Collect great recipes.
- Pass notes during a lecture that has you nearly asleep.
- Redesign something.
- Put the pattern for the socks you're working on in the PDA; then you won't lose it on the plane!
- Keep expense account records then have the computer do the expense account in about two minutes when you get home since the template is already in the computer.

Patti Petit

Saskatchewan, Canada
patti@addmirablewomen.com
www.personaladdcoach.com
ADDmirableWomen: www. addmirablewomen.com

Tip: Estimate time for each task.

With most of my clients, and especially women who are managing households or people with serious time management issues, one of the first things I have them do is estimate how much time they spend doing everything they do. Then they spend a few days actually recording and timing everything from the time they get out of bed in the morning until they go to bed at night. This includes personal hygiene, errands, housecleaning, childcare, etc. This is broken down as specifically as possible (i.e., not housecleaning but vacuuming, dusting, mopping, laundry, dishes, etc.). At the end of a few days, they sit down and compare their estimates with the actual times and see how accurately they had been estimating.

What usually happens is that people's estimates are way off, and they have all sorts of realizations as to why their current routines and perceptions of time are not working for them. From there they are able to better manage the basic tasks and create a routine that better suits their needs. It sounds like a lot of work, but most people end up having a lot of fun doing it, and it's a good introduction to using timers, to using lists, and to getting clients motivated to become more self-aware.

Nancy Ratey, Ed.M., MCC
One of the founders of the AD/HD coaching profession and former President of ADDA (Attention Deficit Disorder Association)
Co-author of *Tales from the Workplace and Coaching College Students with AD/HD: Issues and Answers.*
Wellesley, MA
www.nancyratey.com

Below are two strategies that *help me self-manage,* think in a more "linear way," and help me stay on course and not take so many "detours" (Oh, they can be *soooooo* alluring!):

Tip: Use a "parking lot" for your ideas.
> I keep piles of paper in different places in the house with colored pens next to it. When I think of something I need to do that is not related to my "goal" at the time, I write it on the "parking lot." I collect these at the end of the day and go over them. Many of them are random thoughts or wishes that in the moment I thought were brilliant ideas or things that I felt "pressing." Parking them helps me to curb the urge to act on them, *and* it also helps me to remember important things that I might think of in the moment and don't want to forget.

Tip: Post bulletin boards all over the house.
> I post bulletin boards all over the house and post notes to my self. A huge strategy when packing or preparing to travel or go run errands or prepping for a talk is to use a version of the parking lot idea. I designate a space in my office for the talk, in my room for

the packing, or a space by the door for the errands, and every time something comes to mind regarding that issue, I either write it down and throw it in a basket, open the suitcase, or into a file. Sometimes I start this process three weeks ahead of the event. At least this takes care of the "no brainer" or known aspects of the transition. For example, for travel I list the following: ticket, underwear, running shoes; for errands: car keys, purse, etc. This minimizes the panic to just a few things like: "What errands do I really *need* to run today? (as the pile grows three feet high and blocks the door!)

Miriam Reiss
Business Career Coach
Seattle, WA
www.wisdomcoaching.com

Tip: Tape your bills in your planner so you don't forget to pay them.

A way to pay bills on time is to scotch tape the bill into your planner a day or two before it needs to be mailed out. Seeing it physically in front of you increases the odds that it will go out on time. I recommend regular size planners to my AD/HD clients because they're not lost as easily as PDAs, and if dropped, the results aren't catastrophic.

Harriet Steinberg, RN, MN
Portland, OR
overallorganizer@yahoo.com
www.overallorganizer.com

Tip: Remembering birthdays, etc.—color code them.

I enter all birthdays and anniversaries of friends and family in my calendar in the beginning of the year in red (choose your color). Then at the end of each month, I look at the "reds" for the next month, write the names on a post-it, and stick that in my day planner, so when I go shopping, I know who I need to get cards for. (I hate shopping for cards, so it's less painful if I bunch them together.)

Tip: Use a marker to help match lids for containers.

You know when you're trying to match a plastic lid to a plastic container and you can't find the right fit? I use a permanent marker pen and number the tops and bottoms that fit together. If I have more than one of a same size, then I just use the same number for all of those sizes. It saves a lot of aggravation!

Tips from Professional Organizers
Cindy Eddy
Upper Darby, PA
OrganizerCindy@aol.com
www.organizingteam.com

Tip: Use your Palm Pilot to do scrapbooks and journaling.

Did your child say or do something funny that you always want to remember? Set up a memo in your Palm Pilot with your child's name and keep a running note of all of those funny statements and stories. If your palm has voice recording, even better! Every once in a while, you can print the note and add it to a scrapbook or photo album.

Melody Granger
Lake Charles LA
www.allorganizedforsuccess.com

Tip: Chores—getting kids involved.

I ask children I work with "What would make cleaning more fun?" One five-year-old girl told me, "I get tired and lemonade makes my room clean and makes the bed." The lemonade motivates this little girl. Also, she actually enjoys her two dish nights because this means it is also dessert night. Clean dishes = small dessert. Although you can't lower the sink, it is extremely important to put items they are responsible for within their reach. Basically, if you ask a question, then listen to the answer. Treat them like the individuals they are who have strengths and weaknesses.

Tip: Chores—delegate cleaning according to interest and skills.

As you know, no one likes cleaning, but someone may like to vacuum or sort the mail, so post job descriptions. Make everyone in the household turn in a resume and do an interview! Delegate these tasks to the person most suited for the job. Evaluations and staff meetings are a great way to keep things efficient. Remember, your way may be different than their way of thinking. The end result is what you are looking for. If you give allowances, then pay by the project. Valuable skills can be learned by this "business approach."

Lee Mahla
Owner of Get OrderLee
Sacramento, CA
lee@orderlee.com
www.orderlee.com

Tip: Photograph your kids to help with chores.

To help children with their daily routine, I've taken digital photos of them performing each of the activities they need to complete in order to get out the door in the morning, complete homework, household chores, or the bedtime routine. We printed the digital photos onto sticker paper and then created posters exhibiting the daily routine. The kids enjoyed the process of putting the chart together, but, even more effective than the chart itself was the role playing activity of creating the chart!

Alita Marlowe
Business Oganizer
Marlowe & Associates, Inc.
Farmington Hills MI
www.efficiencyconsultants.com

Tip: Scheduling—time map in planner first.

I'm visual so I have difficulty with a Palm Pilot. I use time mapping in my paper day planner to schedule my appointments. Every Sunday evening I review my week ahead by transferring the appointments into palm software on my desktop (Yes, by hand!). This gives me a heads up about any potential conflicts, gives me a general awareness of my week and allows me to color code my appointments, and print out the five workdays to carry in my portfolio this week. As I plan each day in the morning, it is easy for me to see what's important.

Tip: Reduce kids' clutter using a rolling cart.
For clutter, get a rolling 2 drawer cart from a department store. Use one drawer for each kid. Roll the cart with you and pick up their stuff and put each kid's things in their designated drawer. Roll it into a closet or out of the way. Voila! You now have a clutter free floor. Tell the kids that this is where their stuff is and set up a reward system based on the following: the less time their things are in the cart, the bigger the reward. If the drawer is full when you need to pick up again, there will be a consequence that they won't like.

Tip : Use visualization to prepare for shopping.
I hate grocery shopping. I have organized my pantry according to how accessible things need to be based on how often they are used. Before I grocery shop, I open the pantry door and make a mental snapshot of which shelf isn't stocked appropriately and visualize the aisle in the store in which the product is located. (Only works if you know the arrangement and shop at a regular location). For special one time purchase items, I make a list. If I'm shopping sale items, I circle them with a crayon in the flyer that comes in the mail. And always, always, always, *go alone!*

Sheila McCurdy
Upland, CA
www.clutterstop.com

Tip: Various tips for getting your bills out on time.

The best method of paying bills on time is to pay them when they come in. If you are on a tight budget and must wait for payday, then the bills can be put into a basket, drawer, or shelf that absolutely nothing else goes into or on. For the most part, they will be visible as a reminder. If that reminder becomes unclear, mark on your calendar, in red, "pay bills." Another handy spot for bills is in a product called "EZ Pocket"; it has pockets that are numbered from 1-31. If you stick a bill that's due on the 15th of the month into a pocket that is ten days earlier (the 5th), you can then take the bill out of the pocket and pay it. It is best to make out the check, address the envelope and put a stamp on it so that it is ready to be mailed. The ten days prior to the due date assures you that the bill will get there on time with no late fees. (The EZ Pocket can be bought from my website: www.clutterstop.com and will be shipped directly to a person's home or business.)

Ginger Mitchell & Jennifer Mitchell
Roseburg, OR
www.staywithmehere.com

Tip: Chores—various car care routines.

Unfortunately, routine is the key to having a car that doesn't embarrass you on a regular basis. Until it's time to sell old Betsy, here are some tips for keeping your car sort of clean:

- Choose one day of the week to run your car through the car wash. *Do not* attempt to wash it yourself, at home or otherwise. You'll only do it every week if it's quick and easy.

- Keep *Armour All* wipes and *Windex* wipes in the car. When you're stuck in traffic, you can clean the interior. If you have backseat passengers, put them to work!
- Keep a lint roller in the car to clean the carpet and seats when you are stuck in traffic.
- Find a plastic tote that can hold the miscellaneous items that need to go with you each day (and ideally, to carry the things that should leave the car at the end of the day). The *Rubbermaid Mini Flex 'N Carry*, a plastic tote, works well for this purpose.
- Remember that if you are ever trapped in your car for days due to a freak accident, you will be grateful for the *Cheerios*, popcorn, and the long-lost bottle of water under the seat.

Tip: PDAs and their many uses.

You can use the external keyboard attachment to take notes. We have used these keyboards at large gatherings and have found that the typing enhances concentration just as fidgeting might, and the people sitting nearby have not been distracted by keyboard noise (Targus Stowaway keyboard is fairly quiet). Also, if you are having difficulty paying attention to a lecture or phone conversation, play a game if you find that this helps you to focus on the speaker. Of course, use good judgment as this may be frowned upon in certain settings.

For those who use *Outlook* or another computer program that can be synchronized with a

PDA, a PDA would probably be a wise investment. Calendar pages can be printed out each day or week after making them in sync with your PDA. Use the alarm function to help remind you of important things but here is a word of caution when setting alarms. If an alarm is set for every little thing that needs to happen throughout the day, you will begin to ignore the alarm.

Linda Richards
Gainesville, FL
linda@organizeandmore.net
www.organizeandmore.net

Tip: Palm Pilot's various uses.

1. In the Memo list, put gifts ideas for Christmas and birthdays. Throughout the year, when a loved one says something like, "I'd like ___ someday," secretly write it under their name in your Christmas 2004 memo. If it is clothing, include their size. For fun, make an ongoing wish list for yourself to give to your spouse!

2. Download e-books and read them while waiting in line at the airport or waiting to pick up kids for a carpool. This makes you *happy* when you have delays because then you get to read!

3. Set the alarm chime to remind you of important things such as paying your monthly bills *today* but also set it for fun and/or good mental health things like "Did you take five minutes today to relax and do deep breathing exercises?"

4. Put vacation packing lists in the Memo list.

Have a basic "for any trip" list with items such as underwear, toothbrush, cash, etc. and cut and paste that they're your specialty trip lists. For example, you can have one memo for beach trips that includes items such as suntan lotion, bathing suit, sunglasses, etc. and a different one for skiing trips with items like ski goggles, long underwear, pocket hand warmers, etc. Include reminders such as who will take in the mail and mow the lawn. That way, you'll never forget something important on a trip and only have to do the planning/thinking once!

Ann W. Saunders
Baltimore, MD
aunderannsaunders@aol.com
www.SOSforOrganizing.com

Tip: Time management—work backwards.

For time management, I suggest working backwards. For instance, instead of saying, "I'll set the alarm for 7:00 AM to make a 10:00 AM flight," say "The flight is at 10:00 AM, so I'll need to be at the airport at 8:30 AM. I need to drive there and park, which means I need to leave the house at 7:30 AM, but I need to shower, dress, eat, feed the dog, etc., which usually takes about an hour-and-a-half, which means I need to set the alarm for 6:00 AM! I better add some fudge time, so I'll set the alarm for 5:30."

Tip: To organize clothing, separate by color.

How many times have you reached in the drawer barely awake and pulled out the navy or brown socks, panty hose, or tights when you wanted the black? How about separating the items by color in plastic zip-lock bags with a large label on each? Speaking of labels, when labeling drawers, shelves, or closet space, why not use photos of the items, hand-drawn pictures, or pictures cut out from magazines?

Rebecca Schmidt
Apex, NC
Rebecca@StreamlineMyLife.com
www.StreamlineMyLife.com

Tip: Use a wall-sized calendar to help manage data.

The example I'd like to submit is a past client project I refer to as "The Most Visually Functional Home in the Universe." This particular woman was suffering from the overwhelming amount of organizing products on the market offering to help her color-code, "container-ize" and label everything in her life, so she bought *all* of it. By the time she called me, she was trapped under a pile of these quick fixes and took the first step toward help: admitting she had a problem! After many attempts at different calendar systems, bill systems, mail systems, I needed to be more creative myself. She'd posted birthday cards, upcoming event flyers and other information for the family a six-foot square wall, so this wall became a resource in my mind. The next light bulb worked. We used string to divide the lower (reachable) 5 feet into 5 rows of 7 days...that's right, a calendar! This was a huge calendar where, not only could she post her bills, mail, and events, but she could move her to-do list around and essentially have an inbox full of items on her daily square foot everyday! Of course, we tried this temporarily with string and tape to see if it would work before moving to permanent fixtures. After success, we installed thick, black tape and thumbtacks. We also had to establish some boundary rules for maintenance such as the following: 1) Your day block must be cleared and dealt with before the end of that day, no exceptions! And 2) No papers *outside* the calendar to breed clutter; it's all or nothing.

We went on to store her eight-year-old girl's art on her ceiling, cover a living room wall with old photos previously living in a drawer, and line a large bookshelf with labeled shoeboxes for her new filing system. She still calls at least once a month to tell me about how well she's *still* doing! This is one of my favorite examples of how we as organizers must let go of the 'normal' ideas of being organized to think outside the box to help others on a path you'd never be exposed to otherwise.

Cyndi Seidler
Burbank, CA
cyndi@handygirl.com
www.organized-living.com

Tip: Assign chores to each child.
Assign each child a "hat," i.e., a job to do such as taking out the trash, cleaning up the dishes, setting the table, picking up toys, etc. Teach the child how to do each job and tell them what is expected of them. Let them know that this job is an important function to help you run the house and that their contribution

is valuable and necessary. You can do this for any child of any age over two years old who can speak and walk.

Provide an allowance amount each week for doing this job (e.g., $3/wk) and put the allowance (all in coins such as quarters) in a jar for each child. Each time the task isn't done without asking or reminding, one to two quarters are removed from the jar in front of them. No discussion or arguments should ensue, just do it. Otherwise, the child will not take you seriously and will think that they can just depend on the parent to remind them of doing their jobs.

The child must also perform the job well and may lose quarters if not done to the best of their ability. At the end of the week, the allowance is "paid." A child can earn extra money by doing extra projects, and the money is deposited into the jar for that week. This allows a way for a child to make up for not doing a job. This teaches responsibility and allows a child to contribute and earn rewards for being responsible. The same reward system can be applied to personal hygiene such as bathing, brushing teeth, etc. Money is not deducted for reminders of these activities, especially if the child is very young, but the reward is in the form of bonus points that can be tallied up at the end of the week and turned into extra quarters or some other kind of reward.

221

Peggy G. Umansky, M. Ed
St. Louis, MO
www.itsabout-time.com

Tip: Buddy up with a friend to help you stay focused while studying.

An effective tool for studying when you have focusing issues is to use a friend or acquaintance as a *body double*. This is someone who will sit with you but who does not interact with you unless you have a question. If necessary, give yourself a set number of question cards that you submit to the body double so that you do not continually ask questions. The body double is essentially an anchor, someone to keep you at the table doing your work. Most often, the body double is also doing work. This is also an effective tool for parents to use with children who have attention issues.

Kristin White del Rosso
Pea Organizing Services
Charlotte, NC
Kristin@thepea.com
www.thepea.com

Tip: Palm Pilot—various uses.

Here is some useful information to keep in your Palm Pilot:
- Directions to places you go to a few times a year such as the doctor.
- Favorite websites.
- PIN codes and other important numbers (these can be kept within security walls).

- Date for the car's next oil change
- Monthly breast exam, etc.
- Gift ideas and sizes for family and friends.
- When to pick up items left at the laundry, framing store, etc.
- Where you parked the car at the mall.
- Travel plans and flight schedules.
- Pet records and vet appointments.
- Bank holidays so you'll know when the federal businesses will be closed.

Note: For a directory of coaches, refer to www.addconsults.com and www.add.org.

Chapter 17

...Speaking Words of Wisdom: Top AD/HD Experts Share Their Stories

Over the years, I've read numerous books on AD/HD and have met many, if not most, of the authors of these fine books. I've always been struck with how they managed to write with such apparent ease, in spite of their AD/HD. When I began tackling my own book project, it dawned on me that my readers (and I!) would be interested in hearing their stories. What made them who they are today? How have they managed to become so successful despite their AD/HD?

At the 2004 ADDA (Attention Deficit Disorder Association) conference, authors Sari Solden and Dr. Ned Hallowell took turns interviewing each other. Hearing how they found strength and wisdom in family, friends, faith, and even a first-grade teacher was a profound experience—how despite their own AD/HD, they pressed on to become the influential, impressive people they are today. My goal is to remind you that whether you are an author, athlete, teacher, parent, businesswoman, whatever—having AD/HD does not have to be a roadblock to your success; there are hardships and hurdles, but you can still hit the finish line in spite of AD/HD with support, tools, and treatment. In fact, knowing how

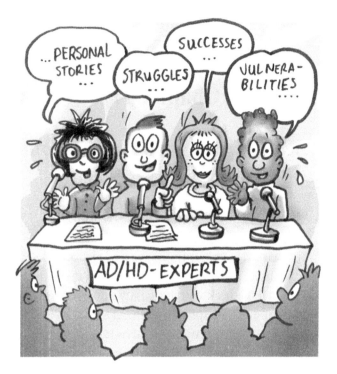

to make AD/HD work to your advantage may even help contribute to your success! Read on to learn what some of the top AD/HD experts in the world have to say about their own struggles and sources of support in response to the following questions (answers may be in random order):

1. Who or what in your life (e.g., family member, teacher, faith, etc.) gave you the confidence and support to help you realize your dreams?
2. What AD/HD "moments" still get in your way, and what have you found that helps you move beyond them—or in spite of them—to become what you are today?
3. What do you know now about yourself that you

226

didn't know ten years ago?

4. Why did you choose to go into the field of AD/HD? What drew you to it?

5. When you write or lecture on AD/HD, what is the most important point you hope your audience comes away with?

Edward (Ned) Hallowell, M.D.
Sudbury, MA
Arlington, MA
www.DrHallowell.com

Co-author of *Driven to Distraction, Answers to Distraction*; author of *Worry: Hope and Help for a Common Condition; When You Worry About the Child You Love: Emotional and Learning Problems in Children; Dare to Forgive; A Walk in the Rain with a Brain* and more. *Delivered from Distraction*, co-authored with John Ratey, M.D., is due out in January, 2005

Do what you love and do it in a way that you love to do it. Be true to who you are. Those have been my watchwords. What I love to do is be with my wife, kids, and friends, so I do a lot of that. My children are like nuclear reactors when it comes to producing hope and joy and meaning in my life. My wife is the classiest act in the world. She is the best, wisest, kindest person I have ever met. I am so lucky she fell in love with me and me with her! My friends are my extended family in many ways. They like me for who I am, which helps me to be true to who I am. I stay away from people who would judge me in negative ways. I stay away from people who do a lot of judging period.

As for work, I love to talk to people about life, so I became a psychiatrist. And I like to help people and see them get what they want from life, so I specialized in an area where I can do that. I love to write, so I write. I write books instead of playing golf. I love to teach so I give lectures around the country. This combination of jobs has given me great variety and tremendous satisfaction. It is very good that I am self-employed. I have always been a lousy employee as I like to do what I want to do when I want to do it. I have worked extremely hard to be able to do this.

My life has been an adventure filled with insecurity and fear but also filled with huge satisfactions. Nothing I have done or will do can match the joy I get from Sue and our three kids, Lucy, Jack, and Tucker. They are my sun and my stars and my everything. Around them I have work, which for me is like serious play.

Of course, I have my problems. I always have to worry about earning enough money, and I have to worry about my relentless personal insecurities, but in the main, I am a deeply happy and very lucky man. I thank God—and Sue—every day.

Sari Solden, M.S., LMFT
Author of *Women with Attention Deficit Disorder* and *Journeys through ADDulthood*
Ann Arbor, MI
www.sarisolden.com

Many people have supported me on the way to realizing my dreams. My husband Dean helped fill in my gaps with his hard work and devotion to my fulfilling my dreams. My publisher, Tim Underwood, gave me the chance to write my book Women with AD/HD, which has been one of the most rewarding and healing experiences of my life. Also, my father, David Shubow, always taught me to "think big."

Disorganization and executive functioning still plague me to a great extent. My self-talk has changed completely, though, in the years since my diagnosis, and so I don't add to the AD/HD difficulties with a barrage of negative self-perceptions. I can separate out my problems from my worth and keep spending as much time as possible in my areas of strength rather than becoming lost in my deficits.

AD/HD is a profound struggle that can't be underestimated, but I have found that it can also be a great asset because it has forced me to search for the truth, depth, and complexity of ideas and to try and discover universal principles. My advice is to learn not just to accept your differences, but to nurture them, develop them, enjoy them, and share them. Ironically, being more open about your uniqueness instead of hiding your differences will help you succeed in the world and to become more intimate with those who are close to you.

I must have been unconsciously driven to find this field. I was working in a minority mental health project and one of my clients had a learning disability so I began looking for ways to help her. As a result, I found myself working with a unique program, counseling adults with learning challenges and surrounded with research on the subject. In the process, I got tested myself and finally understood the roots of some of my own challenges. Eventually, the work I had done in my original area of interest, cross-cultural counseling, formed the basis for my philosophy of counseling adults with AD/HD based on respect for differences.

[My most important message to you with AD/HD is] …to accept the struggle and to transform your losses. To put back the pieces of your life in a new way after diagnosis, not to stay on the surface with treatment but to look for new meaning and a new sense of self. The death of dreams and the goal of getting over who you are lead to much more pain than AD/HD. Meet others like you, get support, and find a unique way to be yourself in the world.

Thom Hartmann
Author of *ADD: A Different Perception; Focus Your Energy; Beyond ADD; ADD Success Stories; The Edison Gene* and many more.
Montpelier, VT
www.thomhartmann.com

[My support system] was a combination of wonderful parents who were willing to reframe AD/HD as "Oh, he's just being a boy and curious" and a few excellent teachers. My grandfather called me and my brothers "the wrecking crew" when we came to visit, but my parents never saw us in that light, and I'm eternally grateful to them for that. In school, there was my second-grade teacher, Mrs. Clark, who on the one hand used to say, "Tommy, an empty wagon always rattles," and, "Even a fish wouldn't get caught if it kept it's mouth shut," yet she accepted me and really wanted to teach me. She kindled in me a love for learning which my parents did, too, but in the context of school.

My biggest challenges are time management and being overly committed, and I can't say I have control over either of those things. The upside, for example, is this year I have published three new books and updated two old books—that's five books total. I write every week and have a daily radio show, and in the midst of this, I have a dozen other projects (radio promotion, guest appearances, etc). So the upside is that I get a lot done because I'm hyperactive and always was; the down side is that a lot doesn't get done nearly as well as it would if I had better time management and didn't over commit. I read my books and think I could have done so much better. It's the story of my life. I think the fact that I'm fairly smart covers up a host of things that otherwise would be obvious. My entire life I have felt and known that I'm not fulfilling my potential. Now at age 53, I've reached a point where I have accepted it.

Twenty five years ago, Louise and I went to a bar in New Hampshire. A big hairy guy named Sweet Pie was singing and playing piano like Jerry Lee Lewis, and in his last set, he played with one hand a series of notes that repeated over and over. He started telling us: "You shouldn't worry what people think of you. Just do your best and say to yourself, 'F*** ' em if they can't take a joke!'" With the other hand, he began taking his clothes off until he was completely naked, all while singing. The whole room was on their feet, shouting encouragement and singing along with him. It was a liberating experience for me. I internalized the message that if you do your best, even if it's not as good as you'd wish you could do but it's an honest effort, then you can accept yourself and get beyond the critical voices in your past.

My son was diagnosed with AD/HD, and we were told that he was "unteachable." At twelve, we were told he was an educational failure. The discovery his AD/HD led to the process of my own self-discovery, as it so often does for other parents. (He's now working on his master's degree at a major university).

[In the end], we have to accept ourselves and our children for who we/they are. If others don't, Sweet Pie has a message for them.

Patricia O. Quinn, M.D.
Director, National Center for Gender Issues and AD/HD
Author of *ADD and the College Student; Re-thinking AD/HD: A guide to Fostering Success in Students with AD/HD at the College Level; Putting on the Brakes; co-author of Understanding Girls with ADHD, and many more.*
Washington, DC
www.ncgiadd.org

Being the oldest girl in a family of five girls gave me great leadership practice bossing them all around. My dad was the one that always let us believe that we could do anything that we wanted. I had no brothers or males to compete with (I went to an all-girls high school and college) and felt girls could do anything they wanted. We shoveled the walks, weeded the gardens, mowed the lawn, and helped build outdoor structures, etc. He encouraged me to venture from the safe path, let me make major decisions, and respected my choices. I also have a saying to sum up how I got this far: "...because no one said I couldn't."

I still tend to hyperfocus and forget important things if I am not working on them directly that moment. (I always used to lock my keys in the car until I got a car that wouldn't let you. I used to forget to pick up my children after I had dropped them off somewhere to play or for practice, and my children grew up and learned to drive themselves!) I also used to have problems with always being ten minutes late for meetings because I thought I would do just one more thing or got distracted as I was starting to leave. Now I set the time I'm going to leave earlier, and I don't let myself do that one last thing. I also try now to aim to be a half hour early. That gives me lots of leeway.

I used to take everything very seriously. I guess I've learned that you shouldn't take yourself or life too seriously. In the grand scheme of things, this is only one decision, one mistake, or one task to complete, and there will be many more. Is this one really that important?

Although my dad, three sisters, and three of my children have AD/HD, I didn't choose this field, it chose me. I was training to be a pediatrician when I became pregnant with my first child. I decided to do a fellowship in child development and needed to conduct original research. I found Dr. Judith Rapoport at Georgetown Medical Center. She had a research grant and needed a fellow. It was research on the treatment of AD/HD, then called MBD or Hyperactivity Syndrome. I fell in love with the work and the 99 boys with AD/HD that I followed for three years, and the rest is history.

[I want people to know that] AD/HD is a very treatable disorder and not a life sentence. Receiving the diagnosis should give them hope that they can now find a path out of the forest.

Kate Kelly, R.N., M.S.N.
Co-author of *You Mean I'm Not Lazy, Stupid or Crazy?!*
and *The ADDed Dimension*
Cincinnati, OH
www.addcoaching.com

My mother always gave me the message that I was special and that I could do anything I put my mind to. Underneath all the struggles with AD/HD, that message was always there in the background. My mom is a really amazing lady. At age 76 she is an icon in the figure skating world because she is still jumping and spinning (not triple jumps, but hey...). Her message is that you are never too old to pursue your dreams.

The AD/HD moments don't really bother me anymore. I laugh and then move on. It has taken 15 years of work to get to this place, and the results more than compensate for the struggle. Most of my AD/HD moments have to do with looking at a task and becoming momentarily overwhelmed. The old tapes start in such as, "You can't do it," "Why bother trying?" etc. Now I catch myself almost immediately, get centered, and move forward. I now know that I am worthy in a way that has nothing to do with accomplishment. The AD/HD community has taught me to put love first. When I do this, all the rest of life falls into place.

I was (and still am) passionate about working with AD/HD after discovering that I had it. I have received so much from the AD/HD community and am delighted to have the opportunity to give back.

I want people to know that we AD/HDers are okay. Better than okay, in fact. AD/HD adults are unique, lovable beings who need to learn self-acceptance and design a life that works with the quirks, so to speak. "How can you be so successful when you have AD/HD?" Years ago, when people asked me this question, I knew what they meant on one level, but on another, I felt like it was a big joke. Yes, I had managed to rack up some very visible successes by writing two well-known books on AD/HD, but I also was well aware of the many things I did poorly or not at all. It just so happens that a gift for using words in a powerful way was strong enough to bypass the effects of AD/HD in that area.

Finally, fifteen years after embarking on my path of recovery from AD/HD, I feel like a real success. That feeling has little to do with the little and larger accomplishments in my life and a lot to do with my attitude. I feel comfortable in my own skin now, AD/HD moments and all. Stopping the mental beatings over my perceived failures has produced a calmer, clearer mind. I am now alert in the present moment.....available for living and learning. In so many areas of life I am really a beginner and am allowing myself to pick up knowledge and skills that other people learned a long time ago..... at my own pac.

There is no longer any need to avoid trying things for fear I will look awkward or stupid because I don't care what "they" think anymore. Freedom from fear is a hard won accomplishment I am extremely proud of. You would probably laugh at my attempts to perform a visual spatial task like putting up a tent. In the past, I would end up standing on the sidelines frozen with confusion and shame while others completed a job that seemed impossible to me. Today I would laugh right along with you. Slowly, I am even getting better at the actual task. Someday, I am convinced that I will master the mysterious skill of tent pitching. For me, it is far more challenging than anything I have to do as an author. In the meantime, I am enjoying the fun of learning without the shame of not having learned it earlier.

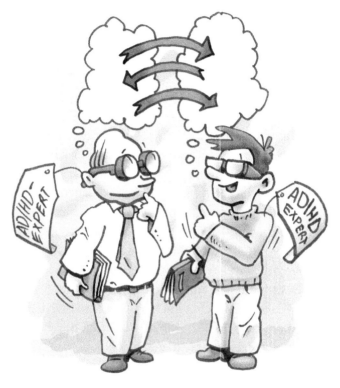

Lynn Weiss, Ph.D.
Author of *Attention Deficit Disorder in Adults: Practical Help and Understanding; ADD and Creativity; ADD on the Job; View from the Cliff: A Course in Achieving Daily Focus* and more.
Central Texas

Because my mental health was compromised growing up, I was forced into some fairly extensive psychotherapy in my 20s. The predominantly helpful Jungian therapist in NYC basically "re-raised me" and taught me that I had value. And he valued "the way my mind worked." All I can say is, "Thank God," terms like Attention Deficit Disorder were not around. He didn't use any diagnostic/medial terms with me so I didn't frame myself in those terms.

Because I have a strong imaginative and creative streak and didn't do particularly well in school (certainly not up to potential), I was drawn to several creative people in my twenties and thirties who supported my sensitivity and dreams. Having been pushed by both society and family to be "educated," my mental health was severely hurt by trying to learn things in linear ways that didn't fit. I did get through a considerable amount of school, though. However, in my twenties, I also found another Jungian who believed in me and was into creative, alternative schooling options (New School in NYC) and crossed disciplines, which fit me well. Finally, through the grace of the Universe, I was able to get my clinical training through an alternative program that was, again, eclectic, multidisciplinary, and hands-on learning. The learning style fit, and I suddenly became "smart." Once I had some skills in my pocket to do something I liked and my own self-belief blossomed, the rest is history. I promise you, none of the traditional environments ever fit me; in fact, they did a lot of damage including family, schooling, and traditional faith (religious) environments.
[In answer to the question, "What ADD "moments" still get in your way...?" my response is that] I don't

accept the wording of "ADD moments." That is patronizing to me. Everyone, including the "so-called normals" (in this culture that usually means someone with a linear brain style) have strengths and weaknesses, i.e., things we do well and easily and things we don't. It *is* hard for me to deal with minutiae (details, especially if they are not connected in a pattern). For example, if I put something on the stove to cook while also working on writing something, if I don't get up the instant the timer goes off so that I can finish a line I'm writing, I will forget that the timer went off. For a creative mind, to stand and focus on a timer going off is so boring as to be discounted. I do not wish to die with time spent "stirring a pot." Compared to writing a thought or creating something, the timer going off is very low on the priority list of my life. So I make a choice (at an unconscious as well as a conscious level) to focus (yes, people like me do focus and quite well) on what interests me.

I also am willing to pay the price of needing to scrub the char off the pot that I have burned because I didn't get up right away. And when I'm tired of doing that (which also takes time from my life), I vow to get up immediately to turn off the pot. This works for a while, but I will revert to my natural way over time. That is just a fact of life and not something I'm going to waste worry time on. I also don't choose to criticize myself or moan about it or even try any harder to do anything about it long term. It's a waste of my time. I can make more money writing than I need to buy a new pot.

The biggest nugget to be shared [in terms of what I've learned over the years] is that I would have given myself permission to be more relaxed about my "natural" way of being and would have spent a lot more time doing what my heart desires. I've discovered that I can be more successful if I do what fits me than if I struggle to be something I'm not or do something that doesn't fit. And, in the long run, I'm happier. I can make trades with others for what else needs to be done. Those trades can be in money, time, skills, or items I make.

I didn't exactly consciously choose [a career in working with ADD individuals], but when one of my sons turned eight and the teacher said, "He could do it if he'd just pay attention," I realized he probably had an ADD style of brain construction. By then the term was around. However, I already knew this child well and knew he had intelligence and perfectly good ways to learn anything. They just weren't the "sit at your desk" and "pay attention to endless detail" type of learning skills. He was/is a kinesthetic learner and because I am, too, we did fine until tradition caught us.

As he went through puberty (the thinking at the time was that ADD went away in puberty), I noticed his ADD style didn't go anywhere. Because I was already willing to question "research" and "experts" and because I was disenchanted, in general, about a lot of the human behavior thinking of the time, I studied what I saw and discovered that I was not much different from him. So I "became an adult with ADD," as it was said then. I found through my radio talk show that many of my listeners identified with me and my son, and there I was, having to write a book to set the record straight. And the rest is history.

[My most important message to individuals with ADD is…] be who you are, do what fits you, and pull away from anyone who tells you differently. Don't consider that you have a problem that needs to be gotten rid of (whether that's through medication, training, or anything else) and find mentors (not necessarily coaches) who have succeeded and are not making their living mentoring. Do what is in your heart and be willing to find ways to make a living and support your family that are non-traditional (non-traditional according to what our culture says is "the right way" to do things).

Nancy Ratey, Ed.M., M.C.C.
Former President of ADDA (Attention Deficit Disorder Association)
Co-author of *Tales from the Workplace* and *Coaching College Students with AD/HD: Issues and Answers*
Wellesley, MA
www.nancyratey.com

I believe my overseas experiences gave me a lot of confidence. I first moved to Brazil at the age of three and then to East Africa at the age of eleven. It was total immersion; I had to learn the language and the culture. Everything was novel. There was no focus on LD or ADD—most everything was hands-on learning, classes were small, there was a lot of one on one help, and most of the ADD attributes in the cultures where I lived were seen as positive and not negative!

Even though learning several languages and understanding life among other cultures taught me how to stand on my own two feet in fierce social settings, these experiences did not make my LD and ADD go away—in some ways, assimilating back to the American schools was much more difficult. I was very advanced socially, but the foundation for basic reading, writing, and math skills was anything but solid, and I knew it. I knew I was very different academically from all the other kids. My self-confidence eroded away quickly like sand against crashing waves.

I would never have ever gotten through those developmentally critical years without my father's support and structure. He taught me "true grit." He taught me resolve. He made me analyze things and would force me to look at things in a different way. This was especially true if I got stuck! If I couldn't get it, whatever "it" was—a problem, a puzzle, a paper or project—on the first, second, or third try, I was expected to continue trying even if it took me to the tenth try or more! It would still be waiting for me the next day with a new query attached to it: "Nancy, what if you looked at the problem from this angle? Or this way?"

My first husband, Joe, fostered the growth of these abilities by believing in me. He believed in me with out restraints. The sky was the limit. He inspired me to reach higher and not to look back or to question how I got there.

Then the true test was surviving the real world. The glue would never have stuck had I not had the opportunity to fail repeatedly. I was very fortunate to have stumbled upon a boss who seemed *blinded* to my disability. He mentored me and believed in me beyond my own capacities. Most importantly, he challenged me to grow.

For me there are still two types of ADD "moments;" both are related. I have a very hard time with transitions of any kind, especially ones that involve travel. Heck, just leaving the house to go three blocks is stressful for me! Presenting is another. Both of these require a lot of linear thinking. I am a very organized person in many ways, however, I don't naturally think in a straight line! And to add insult to injury, I *hate* to make decisions in advance. My mood and my energy pattern the *hour* before any event determines what I pack, wear, and present. This is *incredibly stressful*! I'd like to say that I have it all resolved, but I don't. I've tried every trick in the book. I challenge readers to solve this Rubik's cube of a nightmare I go through. I just know to make sure no one is around me three days prior to a trip. I have also learned to use the same cab company and have for years. They are no longer shocked by my swearing like a sailor and kicking at the luggage upon entering the cab, throwing things all over the back seat as I pack and unpack my bags while on the way to the airport, cursing myself and saying *"I'll never do this again!!*" They also know that by the time I exit the cab, I'll be joking and laughing with them, having already forgotten the trauma from five minutes ago. And before lectures, I've learned to go for a run and walk up and down the stairwells in the hotels before having to review note cards by myself.

I think it is important to know that it is okay to mess up, it's okay to make mistakes, and it's okay to be different. By messing up, we can learn what we want to get better at, meaning, when we make a mistake, look at the opportunities that lie within it. Ask yourself, was this something you really wanted to master? What part(s)? What could you have done differently if you had a chance to do it again? What advice would you give someone else who had messed up in the same way? Give that same advice to yourself. Be gentle. We are definitely our own worst critics. Although my father taught me to be tenacious and was darn proud of all my accomplishments, he also feared that I hung on too tightly and didn't know when to let go. Without a doubt, he took that fear with him to his grave. I regret that. I know now that I have to lighten up, not try so hard, and accept myself for all that I am, for all the extremes—the good days and the bad days—and most of all, I'm learning to let go.

Wilma Fellman, M.Ed., L.P.C.
Author of *Finding a Career That Works for You* and *The Other Me: Poetic Thoughts on ADD for Adults, Kids, and Parents*
West Bloomfield, MI

I was not a superstar in high school. I worked hard and struggled. My grades were average in most things, horrible in math and science, and excellent in writing, English, and public speaking. I had one teacher that took a shine to my writing/speaking style, and she encouraged me (more like bent my arm) to enter a forensic oratory contest. My speech was on fear, and it won at the grade level, school level, and district level and placed third at the state level. I know that my life was altered because of this one incident. I will forever be indebted to Mrs. Gillespie for pushing me when she saw something in me that needed coaxing and nourishing.

[As for my current ADD "moments"], I am still easily overwhelmed. I feel myself shut down when that happens, and I am frozen. My strategy to overcome this is to allow myself the shut-down time and then...to take just one small step to start the productivity going again. The one small step invariably leads to many others (hyperfocusing), and the job gets done. Looking back to the start of this process always amazes me because it always makes me wonder why I felt so overwhelmed in the first place.

I believe that years ago I felt victimized by AD/HD. Now I realize that I have, and have always had, a choice...to lead with my strengths and offset my weaknesses. It's all been in the approach and attitude with me.

I got involved in [learning about ADD] the late '70s because of my son. He was born with a neurological disorder that hospitalized him at the age of six weeks.

His symptoms were alarming: eyes rolling rapidly downward and then staying at half-mast when at rest. He was too young to be lazy! After ten days in the hospital looking for tumors on the optic nerve, epilepsy, etc., he was released with the diagnosis of "Minimal Brain Dysfunction," which was the precursor to AD/HD. This was before it was as prevalent as it is now. Few people knew much about it, and the misconceptions were great. Our whole family struggled with the effects of AD/HD, and I realized then that I had always lived inside an AD/HD body myself. I know firsthand what the struggle feels like, and I understand how confusing this disorder can be. It has been my life to work with people who also struggle with this and to help them find their niche.

I firmly believe that as adults we have choices. We can choose to stand behind our AD/HD and use it as a reason not to struggle (because admittedly, it is a constant struggle), or we can stand in front of our AD/HD and use our strengths and talents to override the challenge. I hope that my work, helping individuals find careers that suit them, accomplishes this.

Peter Jaksa, Ph.D.
Former President of ADDA (Attention Deficit Disorder Association)
Parenting Editor of *ADDitude Magazine*
Author of *25 Stupid Mistakes Parents Make*
ADD Centers of America, LLC
Chicago, IL
www.addcenters.com

My parents grew up in the 1930s in a poor part of Europe and received a third-grade education before they had to go work in the fields. Even so, they always preached the value of education and always provided unquestioned love and faith for me and my brothers and sisters. On a professional level, I was influenced most by a psychology professor at the University of Michigan named Dr. Hoch. Apparently, he saw promise, ability, and a sincere caring about people and recommended graduate school to an impressionable young undergraduate student who didn't see those qualities in himself. He became my professional role model, partly because he also came from humble beginnings, but mostly because he was an incredibly genuine, warm, idealistic person. Looking back now, I'm pretty certain that he was an ADDer, too.

The most frustrating [ongoing ADD] ordeal for me is what I call "living death;" other people commonly refer to it as "paperwork." What I've had to do is set aside half a day during the week, lock myself in my office, put on some music, and do nothing but paperwork. Even then some paperwork gets delayed more than it should, and some people get unhappy with me. Another ongoing problem for me is getting interested and excited in multiple projects and committing to too many things. There is a lot that I want to do but never can find time for.

When Shakespeare wrote "to thine own self be true," he probably wasn't addressing it specifically to ADDers, but boy, was he ever right. Understanding and accepting ourselves is the bedrock of a healthy and happy life. If you have ADD that includes understanding and accepting that part of you. What I have also learned over the past decade or so is that it's far better to pursue goals and dreams than not pursue them, better to take healthy risks than not take them, and better to aim high and challenge yourself than to settle for the expected.

Fresh out of graduate school I started working with children who were labeled "underachievers." They were having problems in school and not performing anywhere near their ability levels. Not surprisingly a *lot* of those kids turned out to be children with ADD. The more I learned about ADD, the more I realized that, hey, it sounded like me! At that point, ADD became a personal interest as well as a professional interest, and I was hooked.

[As far as what I most want to communicate to people about ADD,] I can't pick just one, so how about three main points? The first is that ADD is biology not pathology. What I mean by that is that the biology of ADD is a genetic part of the human race, probably always has been, and probably always will be. It's not a disease you catch or an illness you develop. Yes, it can cause problems for people at times, but there are many people with ADD who are doing just great most of the time. Second, I want people to know that getting a diagnosis of ADD doesn't change who you are — all it does is to make some behaviors more understandable. Some people regard the diagnosis as a label or stigma and start to look at themselves as being different or less of a person because of it. It's not about labels; it's about understanding and acceptance. And third, I want people to know that there is a lot they can do to help themselves if ADD is causing problems in their lives. They can educate themselves about ADD, learn strategies and skills, and take medication if needed. We all have the capacity to learn, find solutions to problems, and make changes we need to make.

Arthur Robin, Ph.D.
Author of *AD/HD in Adolescents,* co-author of *Defiant Teens: A Clinician's Manual for Assessment & Family Intervention,* and *Negotiating Parent-Adolescent Conflict: A Behavioral-Family Systems Approach.*
Professor of Psychiatry and Behavioral Neurosciences at Wayne State University
Detroit, MI

1. Who or what in your life gave you the confidence, support, etc. to help you realize your dreams? (family member, teacher, faith, etc.)
As a child, my mother gave me a great deal of support.
2. What AD/HD "moments" still get in your way and what have you found that
helps you move beyond them—or in spite of them—to become what you are today?
I can't remember names of people I am introduced to at conferences, parties, work, or anywhere else. (My wife) Susan is trained to introduce herself and cause the person to state their name. When I am by myself, I write the

name down on a scrap of paper as soon as is feasible. I still can't get through a meal without getting food on my clothes. Dry cleaners and stain removers get me through this, as well as humor. At home I have my "Italian clothes"— old, red shirts that I wear for eating dishes with tomato sauce.

3. What do you know now about yourself that you didn't know 10 years ago?
Be the "Back-up King." Back up, double check, make extra copies, plan for forgetting, losing, and misplacing because it is going to happen. Be a healthy, obsessive compulsive, coping AD/HDer.

4. Why did you choose to go into the field of AD/HD? What drew you to it?
I was working with children with AD/HD long before I discovered my own AD/HD. The large number of patients with AD/HD I encountered at Children's Hospital (in Detroit) in the early 1980s caused me to learn more about it and eventually specialize in AD/HD.

5. When you write or lecture on AD/HD, what is the most important point you hope your audience comes away with?
Hope that they can cope.

David Giwerc, M.C.C., I.C.F.
President of ADDA (Attention Deficit Disorder Association) www.add.org
Master Certified Coach and the Founder/ President of ADDCA (ADD Coach Academy)
Slingerlands, NY
www.addca.com

My grandmother was a Holocaust survivor. She always made me aware of the strengths I possessed when every one else was looking at my weaknesses. She would never let me fail when I was almost failing math in the third grade. She would wake me up at 4:00 AM each morning, after already drilling me in multiplication tables, and ask me to recite a specific group of multipliers to insure I knew them. I went from almost failing to being one of the best in my class at multiplication. To this day I can do multiplication in my head very quickly.

She also bought me a rocking chair after I had broken two couches from rocking back and forth on the couches while watching TV. I needed to rock and have constant movement so that I could pay attention to the TV. I still have the rocking chair she bought me when I was ten. It was that rocking chair that enabled me to rock my way through studying high school and college classroom lecture notes. I also had to sing my class notes while rocking in order to process and understand the material. She taught me the importance of spending time to make your strengths stronger. She always reminded me that it was my strengths that would get me ahead in life, not my weaknesses.

My perfectionist tendencies [still get in my way today]. [In the past,] I was always so busy worrying about doing things perfectly that I never got things done. I realize that I was trying to perfect the infallible plan that would lead to the perfect result because I was so afraid of not performing well or of failing. Of course, there is no perfect result. I learned a few things from my new awareness and its relationship with my ADD that exacerbated these kinds of tendencies. Perfectionism paralyzes progress. There is no such thing as perfection; there is only excellence. Excellence is the creation of realistic standards that requires the best use of an individual's talents and efforts and the ability to let go of having to achieve [an imagined perfect] result. It means you have to not prejudge the outcome before you even start. You simply do your best based on realistic standards of excellence and then you let go.

[I've learned over the past ten years that] I am a kinesthetic learner who moves around in order to focus, and I need to verbally say what I am paying attention to. I need to hear myself say it or have someone mirror it back to me so that I immediately register and comprehend it. My natural athletic talents that led me to college hoops and a black belt in Budokai karate are what helped me manage my ADD for years without knowing it. Karate has been a tremendous activity for so many reasons such as slowing my brain down so that I can observe and analyze the world around me. It is also the ritual I do before I come up with creative solutions to problems I may be facing or new ideas I want to create. I didn't realize how creative I could be and the natural talents and strengths that were part of my natural personality. I was not able to embrace those then even though people had told me they existed.

[Why was I drawn to working with those with ADD?] I love the underdog. I always have. I can't stand to see people needlessly suffer that are so capable of so much more. [I chose this career because] I didn't want people to have to suffer the way I had. I wanted them to benefit from my experiences and personal stories. When I began coaching entrepreneurs and parents approximately a decade ago, I saw ADDers evolving with amazing leaps, and it was deeply gratifying. Ten years later, it as gratifying now as it was then.

[My most important message for ADDers is] don't let what you can't do get in the way of what you can do. Each individual was put on this earth to live and express his or her inner divinity. People with ADD have a brilliance and radiance that is hidden by the veil of darkness called loneliness and ignorance. Education and community that supports who you are as an individual with character helps lift the negative veil to allow the natural, beautiful, and powerful side of the ADD individual to manifest.

Chapter 18

Savoy Truffle:
SOS Recipes

Is the clock ticking closer to 6:00 PM, and you haven't a clue as to what to make for dinner? Fear not! This is a collection of recipes taken from the archives of my free monthly eNewsletter, ADDitional News. You can sign up on my home page at www.addconsults.com to receive ADDitional news. All these recipes are simple, fast, and very ADD friendly. Enjoy

Tuna Toss
Ingredients:
2 bags salads
1/2 C sour cream
1/2 C mayo
dash of lemon
2 cans tuna
Chinese noodles

Directions: Mix altogether and add noodles last to keep them crunchy.

Eggs in a Bag

Eggs-in-a-Bag is a Girl Scout technique for preparing scrambled eggs exactly the way everyone likes them, without dirtying a skillet or even a plate.

1. Start with quart-size, freezer-style, zip-top bags— one per person.
2. Everyone takes a bag and breaks into it as many eggs as he/she wants to eat.
3. Next, squish the bag to "scramble" the eggs.
4. Then add any of the following: shredded cheese, chopped ham, mushrooms, green pepper, onion, crumbled bacon, or anything else that sounds good.
5. Use a permanent marker to write your name on the bag.
6. Put the bags in a pot of boiling water for several minutes. Once or twice during cooking you may want to remove the bag and, using a cooking mitt, squish the ingredients to distribute the heat evenly.
7. When eggs are the desired firmness, open the bag and enjoy.

Of course, you can always transfer the eggs to a plate if you're willing to wash a dish.

15 Minute BBQ Beef & Rice Dinner

Serves 4

Ingredients:
1 lb. ground beef
1/2 cup chopped onion
1-3/4 cups water

1 cup barbecue sauce
2 cups instant white rice, uncooked
1 cup shredded cheddar cheese
Salt and pepper to taste

Directions:
Brown meat and onion in large skillet; drain. Add water and barbecue sauce to skillet. Bring to boil. Stir in rice; cover. Cook on low heat 5 minutes. Sprinkle with cheese.

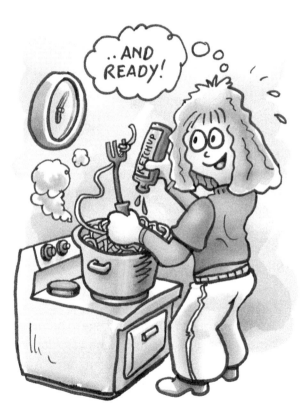

Easy Fish Broil
Ingredients:
4 salmon steaks or fillets
1/2 tsp. dill
1/2 cup real mayonnaise
You can add more ingredients if desired, e.g.,
lemon juice.

Directions:
Spread the mayo evenly over the fish. Sprinkle with the dill weed. Broil for 5-10 minutes until fish is cooked through and topping is golden.

Banana-Sour Cream Crunch Cake
Ingredients:
1 cup sugar
1/2 cup butter
2 eggs
3 mashed bananas
1-2/3 cups all-purpose flour
1/2 tsp. soda
1 tsp. baking powder
4 tbsp. sour cream
1/2 tsp. almond flavoring
Slivered almonds (1/4 - 1/2 cup)

Directions:
Cream sugar and butter. Add eggs and bananas. Combine dry ingredients in a bowl. Alternate dry ingredients and sour cream to mixture. Add flavoring. Beat well. Pour into greased 13" x 9" baking pan. Top with slivered almonds. Bake at 350 for 20-25 minutes or until done. Cut into squares and serve.

Tuna Buns
Serves 5

Ingredients:
1/4 lb. Velveeta cheese, cubed
3 chopped, hard-boiled eggs
1 7 oz can of tuna, flaked
2 tbsp. green peppers, chopped
2 tbsp. onions, chopped
2 tbsp. green relish
1 tbsp. lemon juice
1/2 cup mayonnaise
1 dozen buns

Directions:
Combine all the ingredients, except the buns. Mix well. Cut buns in half. Spread a heaping tablespoon or two of tuna mixture on the bun. Bake covered at 250 degrees for 30 minutes. Makes 10 tuna buns.

Kate and Mackenzie's Favorite Pasta
Ready in: 15 minutes

Note: This recipe was given to me by my mother who is a gifted gourmet cook. Looks like the cooking gene missed a generation because as some of you know, I don't...cook. Luckily, she's passed some of her easier recipes on to me, and I'm sharing this one, which is a favorite of my daughters, Kate and Mackenzie. This one is quick and easy. Good thing, as it has saved the day many times at my house. As a matter of fact, I prepare this almost every week.

Ingredients:
Dry spaghetti noodles (tip: thin noodles cook faster!)
Approx. 1/4 C olive oil
1 large can diced or stewed tomatoes
1-2 garlic cloves, minced (tip: can use prepared, chopped garlic in jar)
Pinch of sugar
Salt to taste
Optional: grated Parmesan cheese

Directions:
Boil water (you can do it!). Add pasta and cook until done. In a separate pot, heat oil. Add garlic and cook on medium heat for about 2 minutes. Add tomatoes and cook on low heat, stirring occasionally until heated through, approximately 5 minutes. Add a pinch of sugar to cut the tartness. Drain pasta, add tomato sauce, and stir. Salt to taste. Can add grated Parmesan cheese if desired

Peach-Cherry Cobbler
Ready in: 20 minutes

Ingredients:
1 can (21 oz.) cherry pie filling
1 package (20 oz.) frozen unsweetened sliced peaches
1 cup biscuit mix
2 tablespoons sugar
1/2 cup milk
1 teaspoon cinnamon sugar
1 pint peach or vanilla ice cream

Directions:
Preheat the oven to 425 degrees F. Butter a 1 1/2-quart baking dish. In a medium saucepan, combine the can of cherry pie filling and the peaches. Bring to a boil over medium heat. Pour into the buttered baking dish. In a small bowl, stir together biscuit mix, sugar, and milk until the biscuit mix is moistened. Spoon over the hot fruit mixture. Sprinkle the topping with cinnamon sugar. Bake 12 to 15 minutes or until the biscuit topping has browned and is baked through. Serve the cobbler from the baking dish and top each serving with a scoop of vanilla or peach ice cream, slightly softened.

Meatballs with Sweet & Sour Sauce
Ingredients:
3 or 4 lbs. ground beef
Grape jelly
Ketchup
Non-stick vegetable spray

Directions:
Use large baking sheets that have sides to catch the grease. Vegetable spray the pans well. Roll the ground beef into balls about the size of walnuts and place 2" apart on the sheets. Bake at 450 degrees until brown and done. Drain on paper towels. Keep warm. In a saucepan, heat equal amounts of ketchup and grape jelly until they are blended well. Use toothpicks to dip the meatballs into the sauce. Delicious with any meatball recipe.

Cherry Topped Lemon Cheesecake Pie
Ingredients:
1 (18 oz.) package cream cheese, softened
1 (14 oz.) can sweetened condensed milk (not evaporated)
1/3 cup lemon juice from concentrate
1 tsp. vanilla extract
1 (6 oz.) ready-made graham cracker crumb pie crust
1 (21 oz.) can cherry pie filling, chilled

Directions:
In large bowl, beat cream cheese until fluffy. Gradually beat in condensed milk until smooth. Stir in lemon juice and vanilla. Pour into crust. Chill at least 3 hours. To serve, top with cherry pie filling. Store covered in refrigerator. Makes 6 to 8 servings.

Candied Yams
Ingredients:
2 large cans of yams
1 cup brown sugar
1 cup pecans
1/2 stick butter, sliced
1 large bag of marshmallows

Directions:
Place yams in baking dish sprinkle with brown sugar and pecans. Put butter slices on top. Bake for 45 minutes in 300 degree oven. When ready to serve, place marshmallows on top and place back in oven till light brown.

Favorite Pot Roast

Serves 4-6
Ingredients:
3-4 lb. beef rump roast
1 tsp. salt
1/4 tsp. seasoned salt
1/4 tsp. seasoned pepper
1/4 tsp. paprika
1 tbsp. instant minced onion
1 C beef bouillon (or 1 cup water plus 1 bouillon cube)

Directions:
Combine salt, seasoned salt, pepper and paprika. Rub all sides of meat with spice mixture. In a crockpot, combine seasoned beef with onion and bouillon. Cover and cook on low for 8-10 hours or until meat is tender. Remove from pot and slice (we like it shredded). If gravy is preferred, thicken juices with flour dissolved in small amount of water after removing meat from the pot.

Note: If desired, vegetables such as potatoes, car-rots, small white onions, celery, or turnips may be added with the bouillon and cooked the same time as the meat.

Jelly Roll Trifle

Ingredients:
1 jelly roll (either homemade or store purchased)
1 package vanilla (or banana) pudding (kind you cook)

Orange juice
1 carton frozen strawberries (about 2 cups) thawed
Whipped cream or Cool Whip

Directions:
Use a glass punch bowl, or other large glass bowl.
Cut the jelly roll into about 1 inch slices and
sprinkle with orange juice. Place the cake around
the bowl and on the bottom. Put a layer of the
cooked pudding on cake, then a layer of the strawberries, another layer of the pudding, and strawberries. Cover all with whipped cream or other
whipped topping. Refrigerate till serving time.

Chicken and Rice Hot Dish
Ingredients:
1 can cream of mushroom soup
1 /2 C regular rice (not instant)
Chicken pieces (enough to cover the casserole dish)

Directions:
Mix a can of cream of mushroom or cream of
something soup (not diluted) with half a cup of
regular rice (not the instant kind). Spread it in the
bottom of a casserole dish. Put pieces of chicken
over the top of it. Bake at 350 degrees for an hour
and a half or so until done. The juice from the
chicken drips down on the rice and makes a yummy
rice dish to serve with the chicken. Amaze your
family! Impress your friends!

Hamburger Packages

Directions:

Make as many hamburger patties as you want to serve and place each one on its own square of aluminum foil. Salt if you are inclined to do so. Put a few rings of raw onion on each patty and quite a few slices of raw potato. Fold up the aluminum foil like you were wrapping a present so it won't leak, put it in a 350 degree oven, and bake for about 45 minutes or until done. No pans to wash!!!

Ham and Broccoli Bake

Serves 6

Ingredients:

12 slices bread, crusts removed
1 1/2 cup diced ham, cooked
2 C frozen chopped broccoli, thawed
5 eggs, lightly beaten
2 1/4 C milk
3/4 tsp. mustard powder
1/4 tsp. onion salt
1/4 tsp. white pepper
3 cups shredded Swiss cheese
Paprika

Directions: Place 6 slices of bread in a greased 9" x 13" square dish. Sprinkle ham and broccoli over the bread and top with the remaining bread. Combine eggs and next four ingredients, stir well, and pour over the bread. Sprinkle with cheese and paprika. Cover and refrigerate up to 24 hours. Bake uncovered at 350 degrees for 45 to 50 minutes or until puffed and golden brown. Serve immediately.

Sweet Potato Bake
Ingredients:
4 to 5 sweet potatoes
3/4 to 1 C brown sugar
2 tbsp. margarine

Directions:
Boil sweet potatoes until tender, drain, and peel.
Then slice in rounds, like coins. Place in deep
baking dish. While sweet potatoes are cooling, boil
together sugar and margarine and enough water to
make a syrup. Then cover your sweet potatoes and
bake in 350 degree oven for 40 min or until
browned a bit.

Spinach and Strawberry Salad
Serves 8

Ingredients:
2 bunches spinach, rinsed and torn into bite-size
pieces
4 C sliced strawberries
1/2 C vegetable oil
1/4 C white wine vinegar
1/2 C white sugar
1/4 tsp. paprika
2 tbsp. sesame seeds
1 tbsp. poppy seeds

Directions:
In a large bowl, toss together the spinach and strawberries. In a medium bowl, whisk together the oil, vinegar, sugar, paprika, sesame seeds, and poppy seeds. Pour over the spinach and strawberries and toss to coat.

Beef Noodle Soup
Ingredients:
1 lb. cubed beef stew meat
1 C chopped onion
1 C chopped celery
1/4 C beef bouillon granules
1/4 tsp. dried parsley
1 pinch ground black pepper
1 C chopped carrots
5 3/4 C water
2 1/2 C frozen egg noodles

Directions:
In a large saucepan over medium high heat, sauté' the stew meat, onion and celery for 5 minutes, or until meat is browned on all sides. Stir in the bouillon, parsley, ground black pepper, carrots, water, and egg noodles. Bring to a boil, reduce heat to low, and simmer for 30 minutes.

Taco Stew
Ready in: 25 minutes

Ingredients:
1 lb. lean ground beef
1 can whole corn, undrained
1 can diced tomatoes with chiles

1 can pinto beans, undrained
1 package taco seasoning mix
1 can tomato soup, undiluted
1 C water
Baked tortilla chips
Monterey Jack cheese, grated

Directions:
Brown beef, drain, and rinse. Combine all ingredients except chips and cheese. Simmer on low until all is warmed. Crumble chips and place in bottom of each bowl. Cover chips with "stew," then sprinkle with cheese.

Oreo Banana Treats
Ready in: 4 hours

Ingredients:
8 Wooden popsicle sticks
4 Bananas—halved crosswise
12 Oreo cookies—finely chopped
2 tbsp. cookie sprinkles
3/4 C peanut butter

Directions:
Insert popsicle sticks into cut end of each banana; set aside. In a medium bowl, mix chopped cookies and sprinkles; set aside. Spread each banana with peanut butter; roll in cookie mixture to coat. Individually wrap coated banana in plastic wrap and freeze until firm. Remove from freezer 10 minutes before serving.

Easy Grilled Salmon
Serves 4

Ready in: 25 minutes (unless you're a klutz with the grill, like me!)
Ingredients:
1 filet (about 2 lbs.) salmon, skin left on
1/2 large onion, finely minced or shredded
2 tbsp. butter
1 tsp. lemon juice
Salt and pepper to taste

Directions:
Mix onion, butter, lemon juice, salt, and pepper in a small sauce pan until the butter melts, so the mixture is spreadable, or you can microwave it for a minute. Place the salmon *flesh* side down on a hot grill; cook about 10 minutes to brown the flesh. Turn the filet over and spread the onion-butter mixture thickly over the top of the filet. Finish cooking for about 10 more minutes, until the skin is crisp and the butter mixture starts to bubble. Serve immediately with hot rice and a green salad.

Easy Greek Salad
Ingredients:
2 (10 ounces) bags ready-to-eat mixed greens
1 (6 oz.) can pitted ripe olives, drained
1/4 C Italian vinaigrette dressing
1 (7 oz.) jar marinated artichoke hearts, undrained
1/4 C crumbled feta cheese
1 small zucchini, thinly sliced

Directions:
Toss greens and olives in a large bowl. Toss with dressing and artichoke hearts with marinade. Sprinkle cheese over salad. Top with zucchini.

Terry's 10 Minute Sweet and Sour Stir Fry
Serves 4

Ready in: 10 minutes

Ingredients:
1 lb. skinless, boneless chicken strips, cut into approximately 1" pieces
2 tbsp. olive oil
1 tsp. chopped garlic
1 box frozen cut broccoli, thawed
1 can regular corn
1 can water chestnuts
1 bottle sweet and sour sauce
1-2 packages boil-in-bag rice

Directions:
Heat oil in large skillet. Add garlic and cook till soft. Add chicken pieces and cook till no longer transparent. Drain fat out of pan. Add broccoli, stirring frequently, about one minute. Add corn and water chestnuts. Add sweet and sour sauce. Stir frequently, covering all ingredients with the sauce. Cook on low heat until heated through, about 5 minutes. Serve with rice
Note: You can substitute almost any frozen or canned vegetables for this, whatever you have on hand.

All In One Tuna Casserole
Serves 4

Ingredients:
1 Envelope Golden Onion Soup Mix
1 1/2 C Milk
10 oz. frozen peas and carrots, thawed
8 oz. medium egg noodles, cooked and drained
6 1/2 oz. tuna, drained and flaked
1/2 C shredded cheddar cheese

Directions:
Preheat oven to 350 degrees F. In large bowl, blend golden onion recipe soup mix with milk; stir in peas, carrots, cooked noodles, and tuna. Turn into greased 2-quart oblong baking dish, then top with cheese. Bake 20 minutes or until bubbling.

Beef Taco Bake
Serves 4

Ingredients:
1 package lean ground beef
1 C tomato soup
1 C salsa
1/2 C milk
1 C shredded cheddar cheese
1/2 C green onion
6-8 flour tortillas cut into 1" pieces

Directions:
Brown beef, drain fat. Add soup, milk, salsa, and half of the cheese. Spoon into shallow baking dish.

Cover and bake at 400 for 30 minutes. Sprinkle with remaining cheese and onions.

Beef Cashew Casserole
Serves 4

Ingredients:
1 lb. hamburger
1 C celery, chopped
1 package egg noodles
salt and pepper
2 cans cream of mushroom or chicken soup
1 medium onion, chopped
3 tbsp. butter
1 C milk
1 C salted cashews

Directions:
Prepare noodles according to directions on package; drain. Brown hamburger, onions, and celery in butter. Mix soup, milk, and seasonings and add to noodles and hamburger mixture. Pour into casserole dish and bake, covered, at 350 degrees for 1 hour. Sprinkle with nuts and bake 10 minutes longer.

Banana Chocolate Pudding
Ingredients:
1 (3.4 oz.) package chocolate instant pudding mix
15 chocolate wafer cookies
3 bananas, sliced
1 C heavy cream

Directions:
Make the pudding according to the package directions and set aside to thicken slightly. Line the
bottom of a serving bowl with cookies and top with
a layer of bananas. Spoon a layer of the pudding
over the bananas. Place another layer of cookies
over the pudding and top with more bananas and
pudding. Continue layering until the cookies,
pudding, and bananas are used. Cover and chill for
at least 30 minutes. In a bowl, using an electric
mixer on high speed, whip the cream until soft
peaks form.

Terry's tip: Use canned whipped cream! Serve
the pudding with the whipped cream on the side.

15 Minute Turkey and Rice Dinner
Serves 4

Ingredients:
1 can cream of chicken soup
1 1/2 C water
1/4 tsp. each paprika and pepper
2 C uncooked minute white rice
2 C cooked turkey or chicken
2 C cooked vegetables (carrots, green beans, peas)

Directions:
Mix soup, water, paprika, and pepper in skillet. Heat
to a boil. Stir in rice, turkey, and vegetables. Cook
over low heat 5 minutes or until done.

Thanksgiving Jello
Ingredients:
1 (6 oz.) package orange Jello
1 can whole cranberries
1/2 can applesauce

Directions:
Mix Jello according to directions; when partially jelled, empty the cranberries and applesauce into the Jello and stir lightly until folded in. Chill until completely set.

Baked Corn
Serves 11

Ingredients:
1 (15.25 oz.) can whole kernel corn, drained
1 (14.75 oz.) can cream-style corn
1 (8 oz.) container sour cream
1 C melted butter
2 eggs, beaten
1 (8.5 oz.) package dry corn muffin mix

Directions:
Preheat oven to 350 degrees F (175 degrees C). Combine the whole-kernel corn, cream-style corn, sour cream, melted butter or margarine, eggs, and corn muffin mix. Mix well and pour into one 9" x 13" baking pan. Bake for 35 to 45 minutes.

Turkey Chinese Casserole
Serves 6

Ingredients:
2 C leftover turkey, diced
2 cans cream of chicken soup
1 can chow mein vegetables, drained
1 can Chinese noodles
1 C diced celery
1 tsp. lemon juice
1/2 C mayonnaise
2 tbsp. onion (optional)

Directions:
Mix all ingredients together and put in greased casserole and bake 1 hour at 350 degrees until bubbly.

Crispy Potato Patties
Ingredients:
2 C mashed potatoes
1 egg, beaten
1 minced onion
1/4 tsp. salt
1/4 tsp. pepper
2-3 tbsp.olive oil

Directions:
Mix together mashed potatoes, beaten egg and onion in a medium bowl. Add salt and pepper and stir. Over medium heat, heat olive oil in a medium size nonstick frying pan. Drop about 1/4 cup of the potato mixture into the frying pan, patting it into 4" circles that are 1/2" thick. Cook until bottom is browned and crisp. Carefully turn the patty over and cook the second side until brown and crisp. Serve with ketchup or salsa.

Ghostly Dessert Cups for Halloween
Serves 15
Ingredients:
3 1/2 C cold milk
2 packages JELL-O Chocolate Pudding, instant, (4-serving size)
1 tub (12 oz.) Cool Whip, thawed
1 package chocolate sandwich cookies, crushed (about 16 oz.)
Mini-chips or other small candies for eyes

Directions:
Pour cold milk into a large bowl; add pudding mixes. Beat with a wire whisk for 2 minutes. Stir in 3 cups of the Cool Whip and half of the cookie crumbs. Spoon 2 tablespoons cookie crumbs and 1/2 cup pudding into 15 individual cups. Top with remaining crumbs. Decorate with remaining whipped topping dropped by spoonful (the ghosts) and make eyes with mini chips.

Ghost Cookies for Halloween
Ingredients:
Nutter Butter cookies
Melted white chocolate
Frosting
Chocolate chips

Directions:
Dip Nutter Butter cookies in white chocolate and let completely dry. Then let the kids decorate the face with cake mate frosting or chocolate chips.

Potato Ghosts for Halloween

Ingredients:
Mashed potatoes
Melted butter

Directions:
Hand sculpt mashed potatoes to look like a ghost.
Place them on an oiled cookie sheet, brushed with
melted butter, and put in the oven to heat and brown
a little. You can serve it with bat shaped meat loaf
(using a bat cookie cutter).

Easy-n-Fast Meatball Minestrone Soup

Serves 6

Ingredients:
2 cans (14.5 oz. each) chicken broth
1 can (14.5 oz.) beef broth
1 bag (1 lb.) frozen mixed vegetables
1 bag (18 oz.) frozen meatballs
1 can (14.5 oz.) stewed tomatoes
1/2 C dried macaroni noodles
1 can (15 oz.) light red kidney beans
1 1/2 t. dried Italian seasoning
6 tbsp. grated Parmesan cheese

Directions:
Pour the chicken and beef broth into a 4.5-quart
Dutch oven or soup pot and begin heating on high.
Add the still-frozen vegetables and meatballs. Add
the tomatoes and macaroni. Cover the pot and bring
it to a boil. This will take about 10 minutes. While
the soup is heating, rinse and drain the kidney beans

and set aside. When the soup comes to a boil, uncover and stir well. (The macaroni sinks to the bottom.) Add the kidney beans and Italian seasoning and reduce the heat to medium. Stir frequently until the macaroni is tender, about 6 to 7 minutes more. Serve at once, garnishing each bowl with 1 tablespoon grated Parmesan cheese.

Quick, Easy-N-Fast Balsamic Glazed Carrots
Serves 2

Ingredients:
2 C baby carrots
1 C chicken broth
2 tbsp. balsamic vinegar
1 tbsp. butter
Salt and pepper to taste

Directions:
Place carrots and broth in small pan and bring to boil. Reduce heat to medium and simmer until carrots are tender and liquid is absorbed, about 20 minutes. Add vinegar and cook over high heat 3 to 5 minutes to glaze. Stir in butter. Season to taste with salt and pepper.

Quick and Easy Peanut Butter Cookies
Ingredients:
1 package golden yellow cake mix
2 eggs
1/2 C shortening
1/2 C peanut butter

Directions:
Blend ingredients in large mixing bowl. Shape into balls. Place on ungreased cookie sheet and flatten with fork. Bake at 375 degrees for 10-12 minutes until golden brown. Don't overcook.

Quick and Easy Seafood Pasta Recipe
Serves 4

Ingredients:
8 oz. small pasta such as elbows, shells, or twists
2 tbsp. butter or margarine
1/2 C chopped leeks, onions or shallots
12 to 14 oz. canned tuna or salmon
1/4 tsp. crushed red pepper flakes
1 tsp. dried basil
2 tbsp. all-purpose flour
2 C milk or cream
1/4 C freshly grated parmesan cheese

Directions:
Cook the pasta, drain, and set aside. Melt butter in a large, nonstick skillet. Add leeks or onions and saute until tender. Add the fish and cook until tender. Sprinkle with red pepper flakes and basil. Stir flour into milk and then stir that mixture into skillet. Cook, stirring occasionally until thickened. Add pasta. Sprinkle with parmesan before serving.

Easy-n-Fast Chicken Strips Recipe
Serves 4

Ingredients:

4 skinless, boneless chicken breasts
1 beaten egg
1 tbsp. dijon mustard
1 tbsp. water
1/4 C flour
3/4 C dry seasoned bread crumbs
2 tbsp. vegetable oil
2 tbsp. butter
1/2 tsp. lemon pepper seasoning
Salt to taste

Directions:
Cut each chicken breast in 6 pieces. In a small bowl, mix together egg, mustard, and water. Add the flour and lemon pepper together on a plate. Place the breadcrumbs on another plate or wax paper. Dip the strips in the flour, then the egg and the breadcrumbs. Repeat until you have coated all the chicken. In a 12" skillet add the oil and butter. Add the chicken and brown on all sides. It should take about 6 minutes. Season with salt. Serve with your choice of dipping sauce or ranch dressing.

Cheesy Crockpot Chicken
Serves 4

Ingredients:
4 to 6 boneless, skinless chicken breasts
1 can condensed cream of chicken soup
1 can condensed Fiesta cheese soup

Directions:
Place chicken breasts in 3-1/2 to 4 quart crockpot.

Pour the undiluted soups over the chicken and stir to combine. Cover crockpot and cook on low 6 to 8 hours until chicken is tender and thoroughly cooked. Serve over rice or noodles.

Shrimp, Tomato, and Rice Salad
Serves 4

Ingredients:
3 C cold cooked rice
1/2 C purchased zesty Italian salad dressing
1/4 tsp. pepper
2 tomatoes, chopped
1 lb. cooked, peeled deveined shrimp

Directions:
Toss together all ingredients. Cover and chill for 30 minutes to blend flavors.

Waldorf Chicken Salad Sandwich
Serves 4

Ingredients:
4 Kaiser rolls, cut in half
1 C deli chicken salad
12 very thin apple slices
4 slices cheddar cheese

Directions:
Layer bottom half of each roll with salad, 3 apple slices, and 1 cheese slice. Top with tops of rolls.

Black Bean Lasagna
Serves 10

Ingredients:
1 15 oz. can black beans, drained and rinsed
1 26 oz. can crushed tomatoes, undrained
2 chopped onions
2 cloves garlic, minced
1 chopped green bell pepper
1-1/2 C salsa
1 tsp. chili powder
1/2 tsp. cumin
2 C light ricotta cheese
1 egg
1/2 C grated parmesan cheese
10 uncooked lasagna noodles
2 C shredded Co-jack cheese

Directions:
In large bowl, combine drained beans, tomatoes, onions, garlic, bell pepper, salsa, chili powder, and cumin; mix well. In small bowl, combine ricotta cheese, egg, and parmesan cheese; beat until combined. Spread 1 cup of the tomato mixture in the bottom of a 13" x 9" glass baking dish. Top with half of the noodles, overlapping slightly. Top with half of remaining tomato mixture. Spoon ricotta mixture over the top, spreading carefully. Sprinkle with 1/2 cup Co-jack cheese. Layer remaining noodles and tomato mixture over the casserole. Top with remaining Co-jack cheese. Spray sheet of foil with cooking spray, and cover baking dish with foil, sprayed side down. Bake at 350 degrees for 50-65 minutes or until noodles are tender. Uncover and

bake 10 minutes longer until casserole is bubbling.
Let stand 15 minutes before serving.

Make Ahead Scrambled Eggs
Serves 8

Ingredients:
12 eggs
1/2 C cream
1/4 tsp. salt
1/4 tsp. pepper
2 tbsp. butter
8 oz. sour cream
1 C shredded cheddar cheese

Directions:
Beat eggs with cream in a large bowl. Stir in salt
and pepper. Melt butter in large skillet over medium heat. Pour eggs into skillet and cook, stirring
frequently, until eggs are scrambled and set. Remove pan from heat and stir in sour cream. Spread
eggs into a greased 12" x 7" glass baking dish.
Sprinkle with cheese. Cover tightly and refrigerate
overnight. When ready to eat, preheat oven to 300
degrees. Uncover the baking dish and bake for 15
to 20 minutes or until cheese is melted and eggs are
hot.

Sour Cream Ham over Potatoes
Ingredients:
4 baking potatoes, scrubbed
1/4 C butter
2 C sliced fresh mushrooms

1/4 C chopped green onions
1 C diced deli ham
1/4 C sour cream
3 tsp. honey mustard
1 C shredded cheddar cheese

Directions:
Cook potatoes in microwave until soft; set aside. In microwave container, combine butter, mushrooms, and green onion. Microwave on high for 2-4 minutes until mushrooms are tender. Add ham and microwave on high for 1-2 minutes until thoroughly heated. Stir in sour cream and mustard. Cut potatoes in half lengthwise and mash slightly with fork. Spoon ham mixture over each potato half and sprinkle with cheese. Microwave on high for 2-3 minutes until cheese is melted.

Old-Fashioned Goulash
Serves 6

Ingredients:
3 C rotini pasta
1 lb. ground beef
2 chopped onions
10-oz. can condensed tomato soup
2 14-oz. cans diced tomatoes with garlic, undrained

Directions:
Preheat oven to 350 degrees. Cook pasta according to package directions and drain. Meanwhile, cook ground beef and onion until meat is browned and onion is tender, stirring to break up meat. Drain well. Add soup and diced tomatoes and cook for 3-

5 minutes until blended, stirring frquently. Add
pasta and pour into 3 quart glass casserole. Bake at
350 degrees for 40-50 minutes until bubbly and hot.

Five-Minute Fudge
Serves 20

Ingredients
2 tbsp. butter
2/3 C evaporated milk
1 2/3 C sugar
1/2 tsp. salt
2 C miniature marshmallows
1 1/2 C semi-sweet chocolate chips
1 tsp. vanilla
1/2 C chopped nuts (opt)

Directions:
Combine first four ingredients in a heavy saucepan.
Cook over medium heat and bring to a boil. Cook
4-5 minutes, stirring constantly. (Start timing when
mixture starts to 'bubble' around edges of pan.)
Remove from heat. Add marshmallows, chocolate
chips and vanilla. Stir until melted. Add nuts. Pour
into an 8" square, buttered pan. Cool. Cut into
squares.

Quick and Easy Chicken
Serves 4

Ingredients:
2 tablespoons olive oil
1 onion, chopped

4 skinless, boneless chicken breast halves
3 tablespoons ketchup
2 tablespoons soy sauce
3 tablespoons white sugar
2 tablespoons lemon juice
1 teaspoon ground black pepper

Directions:
Saute onion in oil until translucent.
Add chicken, and brown lightly.
Combine ketchup, soy sauce, sugar, lemon juice, and pepper; mix well. Pour over chicken, and bring to a boil. Cover, reduce heat, and simmer for 25 to 35 minutes.

Chapter 19

Do You Want to Know a Secret? Books, Tapes, Web Sites, Newsletters, and More

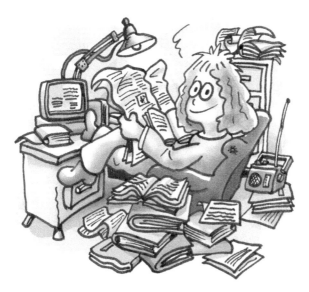

Books and Video Tapes

Girls and Women with AD/HD

Adamec, C. (2000). *Moms with ADD: A self-help manual*. Dallas, TX: Taylor Trade Publishing.

Nadeau, K., Littman, E., & Quinn, P. (1999). *Understand-*

ing girls with AD/HD. Silver Springs, MD: Advantage Books.

Nadeau, K., & Quinn, P. (Ed.). (2002). *Understanding women with AD/HD*. Silver Springs, MD: Advantage Books.

Solden, S. (1995). *Women with attention deficit disorder*. Grass Valley, CA: Underwood Books.

Children and Teens with AD/HD

Barkley, R. A. (1995). *Taking charge of ADHD*. New York: Guilford Press.

Dendy, C. (1995). *Teenagers with ADD: A parents' guide*. Bethesda, MD: Woodbine House.

Goldstein, S., & Goldstein, M. (1998). *Managing attention deficit hyperactivity disorder in children*. New York: John Wiley & Sons, Inc.

Greenbaum, J. & Markel, G. (2001). *Helping adolescents with AD/HD and learning disabilities*. Des Moines, IA: Prentice Hall.

Phelan, T. (1995). *1-2-3 magic*. Glen Ellyn, IL: Child Management, Inc.

Rief, S. (2003). *The AD/HD book of lists*. Hoboken, NJ: Jossey-Bass.

Robin, A. (2002). *Negotiating parent-adolescent conflict: A behavioral-family systems approach*. New York: The Guildford Press.

General Books on AD/HD

Amen, D. G. (1995). *Windows into the A.D.D. mind: Understanding and treating attention deficit disorders in the everyday lives of children, adolescents and adults*. Fairfield, CA: MindWorks Press.

Amen, D. G. (2001). *Healing ADD: The breakthrough*

program that allows you to see and heal the 6 types of ADD. New York: G. P. Putnam & Sons.

Barkley, R. A. (1997). *AD/HD and the nature of self-control.* New York: Guilford Press.

Barkley, R. A. (1998). *Attention deficit hyperactivity disorder: A handbook for diagnosis and treatment.* (2nd ed.). New York: Guilford Press.

Bramer, J. S. (1996). *Succeeding in college with attention deficit disorders.* Plantation, FL: Specialty Press, Inc.

Fellman, W. R. (1997). *The other me: Poetic thoughts on ADD for adults, kids and parents.* Plantation, FL: Specialty Press, Inc.

Fowler, R. (1995). *Honey, are you listening?* Nashville, TN: Thomas Nelson Publishers.

Hallowell, E., & Ratey, J. (1994). *Driven to distraction.* New York: Pantheon Books.

Hallowell, E., & Ratey, J. (1995). *Answers to distraction.* New York: Pantheon Books.

Halverstadt, J. (1998). *A.D.D. and romance: Finding fulfillment in love, sex, and relationships.* Dallas: Taylor Publishing Company.

Hartmann, T., & Ratey, J. (1995). *ADD success stories: A guide to fulfillment for families with attention deficit disorder: Maps, guidebooks, and travelogues for hunters in this farmer's world.* Grass Valley, CA: Underwood Books.

Hartmann, T. (1997). *Attention deficit disorder: A different perception.* Grass Valley, CA: Underwood Books.

Hartmann, T. (1998). *Healing ADD: Simple exercise that will change your daily life.* Grass Valley, CA.: Underwood Books.

Hartmann, T. (2003). *The Edison gene: AD/HD and the gift*

of the hunter child. Rochester, VT: Park Street Press.

Ingersoll, B. (1998). *Daredevils and daydreamers.* New York: Doubleday.

Kelly, K. & Ramundo, P. (1995). *You mean I'm not lazy, stupid, or crazy?!* Cincinnati, OH: Scribner.

Kelly, K. & Ramundo, P. (1997). *The ADDed dimension: Everyday advice for adults with ADD.* New York: Scribner.

Latham, P., & Latham, P. (1992). *Attention deficit disorder and the law: A guide for advocates.* Washington, DC: JKL Communications.

Mate', G. (1999). *Scattered: How attention deficit disorder originates and what you can do about it.* New York: Dutton.

Murphey, K. R., & Levert, S. (1995). *Out of the fog: Treatment options and coping strategies for adult attention deficit disorder.* New York: Hyperion/Skylight Press.

Nadeau, K. (Ed.) (1995). *A comprehensive guide to attention deficit disorder in adults.* New York: Brunner/ Mazel Trade.

Nadeau, K. (1996). *ADD in the workplace: Choices, changes and challenges.* New York: Brunner/Mazel Trade.

Nadeau, K. (1996). *Adventures in fast forward: Life, love and work for the ADD adult.* New York: Brunner/ Mazel Trade.

Novotni, M., & Peterson, R. (1999). *What does everyone know that I don't?* Plantation, FL: Specialty Press, Inc.

Quinn, P., Ratey, N., & Maitlan, T. (2000). *Coaching college students with AD/HD: Issues & answers.*

Betheseda, MD: Advantage Books.

Richardson, W. (1997). *The link between ADD and addiction: Getting the help you deserve.* Colorado Springs, CO: Pinon Press.

Solden, S. (2002). *Journeys through ADDulthood.* New York: Walker & Company.

Weiss, L. (1992). *Attention deficit disorder in adults: Practical help and understanding.* Dallas: Taylor Publishing.

Weiss, L. (1995). *ADD and creativity: Tapping your inner muse.* Dallas: Taylor Trade Publishing.

Weiss, L. (1996). *ADD on the job.* Dallas: Taylor Trade Publishing.

Weiss, L. (2001). *View from the cliff.* Dallas: Taylor Trade Publishing.

Wender, P. (1995). *Attention-deficit hyperactivity disorder in adults.* New York: Oxford University Press.

Whiteman, T., & Novotni, M. (1995). *Adult ADD: A reader-friendly guide to identifying, understanding, and treating adult attention deficit disorder.* Colorado Springs, CO: Pinion Press.

Organizing

Aslett, D. (1995). *Clutter free, finally and forever.* Cincinatti, OH: Betterway Publishers.

Culp, S. (1989). *How to conquer clutter.* Cincinnati, OH: F & W Publications.

Felton, S. (2000). *The new messies manual.* Grand Rapids, MI: Fleming N. Revell.

Glovinsky, C. (2002). *One thing at a time: 100 simple ways to live clutter-free every day.* New York, NY: St. Martin's Griffin.

Glovinsky, C. (2004). *Making peace with the things in your life.* New York: St. Martin's Griffin.

Hempshill, B. *Taming the paper tiger.* (1997). Washington, DC: Kiplinger Books.

Kolberg, J. (1999). *Conquering chronic disorganization.* DeCatur, GA: Squall Press.

Kolberg, J. & Nadeau, K. (2002). *ADD-friendly ways to get organized.* New York: Taylor and Francis.

Lehmkuhl, D. (1993): *Organizing for the creative person.* New York: Crown Trade Paperbacks.

Morgenstern, J. (1998). *Organizing from the inside out.* New York: Henry Holt & Company, Inc.

Morgenstern J. (2000). *Time management from the inside out.* New York: Henry Holt & Company, Inc.

Schlenger, S. & Roesch, R. (1999). *How to be organized in spite of yourself.* New York: Penguin.

Of General Interest

Aron, E. (1997). *The highly sensitive person: How to thrive when the world overwhelms you.* New York: Broadway Books.

Covey, S. (1989). *The 7 habits of highly effective people.* New York: Simon & Schuster.

Fellman, W. R. (2000). *Finding a career that works for you.* Plantation, FL: Specialty Press, Inc.

Hallowell, E. (2001). *Human moments: How to find meaning and love in your everyday life.* Deerfield Beach, FL: Health Communications, Inc.

Hallowell, E. (2004). *Dare to forgive.* Deerfield Beach, FL: Health Communications, Inc.

Heller, S. (2003). *Too loud, too bright, too fast, too tight: What to do if you are sensory defensive in an over-stimulating world.* New York: HarperCollins Publishers.

Jaksa, P. (1999). *25 stupid mistakes parents make.* Los Angeles: Lowell and House.

Lerner, H. (1985). *The dance of anger.* New York: HarperCollins.

Lerner, H. (1989). *The dance of intimacy.* New York: Harper & Row.

Lerner, H. (2001). *The dance of connection: How to talk to someone when you're mad, hurt, scared, frustrated, insulted, betrayed, or desperate.* New York: Harper & Row.

Payson, E. (2002). *The wizard of oz and other narcissists.* Royal Oak, MI: Julian Day Publications.

Ratey, J. (2001). *A user's guide to the brain.* New York: Pantheon Books.

Ratey, J., & Johnson, C. (1997) *Shadow syndromes.* New York: Pantheon Books.

Viorst, J. (1986). *Necessary losses: The loves, illusions, dependencies, and impossible expectations that all of us have to give up in order to grow.* New York: Ballantine Books.

Video Tapes

ADD Coach Academy (Producer). (2000) *David Giwerc: Me, my ADD coach, and I* [Videotape]. (Available at www.addca.com or www.myADDstore.com)

Amen, D. (Producer). (1995). *A.D.D. in intimate relationships: Problems and solutions for couples affected by A.D.D.,* [Videotape]. (Available from MindWorks Press, www.mindworkspress.com)

Feldman, E. (Producer), & Kay, T. (Director). (1999). *Outside in: A look at adults with Attention Deficit Disorder* [Videotape]. (Available from the Attention Deficit Disorder Association, www.add.org)

Solden, S. (Producer). (1995). *Women with attention deficit disorder*. [Videotape]. (Available at www.sarisolden.com)

Media
Web Sites, Newsletters, Mailing Lists, Magazines, and Catalogs

Web Sites of Interest to Women with AD/HD
ADDmirableWomen

www.addmirablewomen.com

ADDmirableWomen is an online support community for women with AD/HD, offering information, resources, forums, and a variety of email-based support groups.

ADDvance

www.addvance.com

Dr. Patricia Quinn's and Dr. Kathleen Nadeau's online resource for women with AD/HD, offering articles, resources, and more.

National Center for Gender Issues and AD/HD

www.ncgiadd.com

Non-profit organization promoting awareness, advocacy, and research on AD/HD in women and girls. Web site offers resources, articles, and newsletter.

Sari Solden

www.sarisolden.com

Web site of Sari Solden, bestselling author of *Women with Attention Deficit Disorder*; Q and A with Sari, forums, and a screening checklist for women.

Web Sites with General AD/HD Information and Products

ADD at About.com

> www.add.about.com
>
> Forums, articles, and updates on AD/HD.

ADD Consults

> www.addconsults.com
>
> Terry Matlen's one-stop-shop for all things AD/HD: online consultations, free support groups, online conferences, directory of professionals, coaches, articles, store, free eNewsletter, and more.

ADDers.org (International resources)

> www.adders.org
>
> An international site listing support groups, articles, research updates, and forums.

ADD Forums

> www.addforums.com
>
> Lots of great forum discussions; a great place to find support.

ADD Resources

> www.addresources.org
>
> Non-profit organization offering a lending library, conferences, newsletter, and articles. *(See "Organizations.")*

AD/HD Information and Support Services ADDISS (UK)

> www.addiss.co.uk *(See "Organizations").*

AD/HD News

> www.adhdnews.com
>
> Articles, resources, and support.

Attention Deficit Disorder Association (ADDA)

> www.add.org
>
> Members enjoy many resources plus a great quarterly newsletter.

Children and Adults with AD/HD (CHADD)
> www.chadd.org
> Find support groups near you plus other great resources.

LD Online
> www.ldonline.org/
> Resources and information on learning disabilities.

Living with ADD
> www.livingwithadd.com
> Articles, stories, and tips.

My ADD Store
> www.myADDstore.com
> Terry Matlen's site has hundreds of products to make life with AD/HD just a bit easier: clothes for the hypersensitive (tagless t-shirts, seamless socks, flannel clothes); sensory items to help calm you down, organizing products, fidgets, books, magazines, last minute gifts, parenting tools, and much more. www.myADDstore.com Note: *(See Product Section on the following pages for a brief description of a number of products.)*

myADHD
> www.myadhd.com
> Tools to connect doctors, parents, teachers, and adults.

National Institute of Mental Health (NIMH) AD/HD
> www.nimh.nih.gov/healthinformation/adhdmenu.cfm
> Information on AD/HD, articles, and research updates.

National Resource Center for AD/HD
> www.help4adhd.org/
> National clearinghouse of information and resources.

Schwab Learning Foundation
> www.schwablearning.org
> Information on AD/HD and kids, dealing with
> schools, and a parent message board.

Newsletters, Catalogs, Magazines, and Forums

ADDitional News
> www.addconsults.com
> Free news publication provided by Terry Matlen's
> ADD Consults sent via eMail. Forums at
> www.addconsults.com/tforum.

ADD International Professionals
> http://health.groups.yahoo.com/group/ADD-Inter
> national/
> International list for clinicians and researchers who
> have master's level degrees and above.

ADDitude Magazine
> www.additudemag.com
> Quarterly print magazine with articles on AD/HD,
> available at bookstores or at their Web site.

ADD Professionals
> http://health.groups.yahoo.com/group/
> ADDprofessionals
> An AD/HD professionals' mailing list (clinicians,
> coaches, educators, and advocates).

ADDvisor
> www.ADDvisor.com
> Newsletter sent via email with articles and re-
> sources on AD/HD.

ADD Warehouse
> www.addwarehouse.com
> Catalogue of books, magazines, tapes, and more on

AD/HD.

800-233-9273

The AD/HD Report

800-365-7006

Print newsletter with the latest in AD/HD research.

ATTENTION

www.chadd.org

Print newsletter mailed quarterly to CHADD members.

Attention Research Update

www.helpforadd.com

Email newsletter that reviews recently published AD/HD studies.

FOCUS

www.add.org

Print newsletter mailed quarterly to ADDA members.

Online Mailing Lists

ADD Bulletin Board

www.health.groups.yahoo.com/group/
ADHD_Bulletin_Board

Updates on AD/HD research, general information, and resources.

ADDMirable Women

www.health.groups.yahoo.com/group/
addmirablewomen

Support for women with AD/HD.

ADDwomen

www.health.groups.yahoo.com/group/addwomen

Support for women with AD/HD.

Fly Lady

www.flylady.net

Emails sent daily with organizing tips.
Organizer Lady
>www.groups.yahoo.com/group/The-Organizer-Lady
>Emails sent daily with organizing tips.

MSN Groups
>www.groups.msn.com/ (search using "ad/hd" or
>"attention deficit")
>Large listing of AD/HD groups.

YahooGroups
>www.groups.yahoo.com/ (search with key word
>"attention deficit disorder")
>>Large listing of AD/HD groups.

Miscellaneous Resources
FREE *ADD eBook*
>www.pediatricneurology.com/adhd.htm

Support

Chat Rooms and Hotlines
ADD Consults
>www.addconsults.com/digichat
>ADD Consults offers online live support chats for
>AD/HD women only every Thursday at 9:30 PM
>EST. There are other groups for men *and* women;
>please check the schedule at the URL above.

AOL

Keyword "AD/HD"

Messies Anonymous
>www.messies.com

Note: Some *Yahoo* mailing lists have associated chats. Check by going to www.yahoogroups.com and searching with keyword "AD/HD."

Organizations

ADA Information Line (U.S. Dept. of Justice)
  800-514-0301

ADD Resources
  www.addresources.org
  Non-profit organization offering lending library, conferences, newsletter, and articles.

AD/HD Information and Support Services ADDISS (UK)
  www.addiss.co.uk

Attention Deficit Disorder Association (ADDA)
  P.O. Box 543
  Pottstown, PA 19464
  Phone: 484-945-2101
  www.add.org

Children and Adults with Attention Deficit/Hyperactivity Disorder (CHADD)
  8181 Professional Place
  Suite 201
  Landover, MD 20785
  (800) 233-4050
  www.chadd.org

EEOC (Equal Employment Opportunity Commission)
  • for ADA documents: 800-669-3362
  • for ADA questions: 800-669-4000

Job Accommodation Network
  800-526-7234

Learning Disability Association of America (LDA)
  4156 Library Road
  Pittsburgh, PA 15234

(412) 341-1515

www.ldanatl.org

National Association for Professional Organizers (NAPO)
(847) 375-4746

www.napo.net

National Center for Gender Issues and ADHD
1001 Spring Street, Suite 206
Silver Spring, MD 20910
(202) 966-1561

www.ncgiadd.org

National Study Group on the Chronically Disorganized
916-962-6227

www.nsgcd.org/

President's Committee on Employment of People with Disabilities
202-376-6200

U.S. Department of Education Regional of People with Disabilities
800-949-4232

Web Sites of the AD/HD Experts

Dr. Daniel Amen
www.amenclinic.com

Dr. Sam Goldstein
www.samgoldstein.com

Dr. Ned Hallowell
www.drhallowell.com

Thom Hartmann
www.thomhartmann.com

Dr. Peter Jaksa
www.addcenters.com

Kate Kelly
    www.addcoaching.com
Dr. John Ratey
    www.johnratey.com
Nancy Ratey
    www.nancyratey.com
Wendy Richardson
    ww.addandaddiction.com
Sari Solden
    www.sarisolden.com

Coaching Web Sites

ADD Coach Academy
    www.addcoachacademy.com
ADD Consults Coach Directory
    www.addconsults.com
American Coaching Association
    www.americoach.org
Optimal Functioning Institute
    www.addcoach.com

Web Sites for Help with Disorganization

Conveniencenet.com
    www.conveniencenet.com
Get Organized Now!
    www.getorganizednow.com
List Organizer
    www.listorganizer.com
National Association for Professional Organizers (NAPO)
    (847) 375-4746
    www.napo.net
National Study Group on the Chronically Disorganized
    1-916-962-6227

www.nsgcd.org
Online Organizing.com
www.onlineorganizing.com
Organize Tips
www.organizetips.com
Organized-Mom
www.organized-mom.com
Sidetracked Home Executives
www.shesintouch.com
Sort-It
www.123sortit.com

Miscellaneous Web Sites
All Kinds of Minds
www.allkindsofminds.org
Job Accommodation Network
www.jan.wvu.edu/
Job Applicants and the Americans with Disabilities Act
www.eeoc.gov/facts/jobapplicant.html
Mind Tools
www.mindtools.com
Reed Martin
www.reedmartin.com
Special education law.
U.S. Equal Employment Opportunity Commission
www.eeoc.gov/
Wright's Law
www.wrightslaw.com

Products
Those products with an * can be found on the web at :
www.myADDstore.com

Organizing Products

Car Organizer

> To keep your car tidy, use the *Car Organizer.* It has a flip-top tray lid which holds food or car supplies. The corner pocket holds mail and notes, and a clipboard holds pad, maps, or papers. If you're in your car a lot and need access to your "stuff," this is a great way to have things handy in your front seat without messing up your car.

Couponizer

> Do you have store coupons in stacks around your house, or stuffed in your pockets and purse? The *Couponizer* solves that problem by helping you to organize, store, and access coupons while you shop.

Don't Forget Hanging Organizer

> The *Don't Forget Hanging Organizer* (it actually says "Don't forget" at the top!) has labeled pouches for you to store things like your keys, glasses, and coupons plus unlabeled pouches for your other items you don't want to leave home without.

EZ Pocket

> *EZ Pocket* keeps track of bills, appointments, invitations, and more. The canvas hanger has large pockets that you can organize by date or project. You can order this at the following Web site: www.ezpocket.com

Gift Wrap Organizer

> The *Gift Wrap Organizer* solves the problem of not

being able to find your wrapping paper, tape, and scissors and prevents clutter by holding up to 14 rolls of paper. I like this because you can close it up and store it nicely in a closet.

Hanging Bill Organizer

The *Hanging Bill Organizer* is similar to the *Don't Forget Hanging Organizer* above, but this keeps track of your incoming and outgoing bills. Because it's a visual reminder and storage unit, you'll be less apt to throw your bills in piles. It even comes with a pouch for stamps and has text at the top that says "You've Got Bills." Very clever!

Jewelry Organizer

The *Jewelry Organizer* has tons of pouches to hold your jewelry, which can then be hung in your closet for easy storage and viewing. No more tangled up necklaces and earrings dumped into a bottomless jewelry box; now it's all easy to put away and retrieve.

Magazine Bin with Pockets

Lillian Vernon's *Magazine Bin with Pockets* is an attractive way to solve the piles of magazines problem. It can be folded, too, for easy storage. There are also outside pockets to hold other "stuff." You can use this for your kids coloring books and crayons, too.

Magellan Meridian Gold GPS Receiver

Stop getting lost! The *Magellan Meridian Gold GPS Receiver* works in your car or on hiking trails and guides you to wherever you need to go.

* *Now You Can Find It*

> *Now You Can Find It* solves the problem of lost keys, PDAs, glasses, and anything else that finds its way to the darkest holes of your house. Just press a button, and the lost item beeps so you can retrieve it.

*Pantry Organizer

> The *Pantry Organizer* is a great way to keep your cans and spices easily stored and tidy. It has three steps and is expandable.

*Purseket

> Dig in your garden, not your purse! The *Purseket* is an organizer for your purse. It comes in various sizes and is basically a strip of pockets that, when inserted into your purse, conforms to its shape. All your items can be stored in the pockets, and the middle pocket is left open for larger objects like your wallet. No more digging in the bottom of your purse!

**School Days Organizer*

> Keep your child's school work and art projects safe and organized with the *School Days Organizer*. The 6-drawer chest holds items from preschool to grade 6, and it comes with a book and envelopes to hold even more school related memories.

* *Student Locker File*

> Organize your child's school locker with the *Student Locker File*. Five colorful, removable pockets divide school subjects. They cascade down for instant access and can hang from the built-in hook.

The clear front pocket displays pictures or a class schedule. Includes a clipboard to hold loose papers. Folds into its own compact case for carrying in a backpack.

Teddy Hammock

Take hold of your child's massive doll, teddy bear, or Beanie collection with the *Teddy Hammock*. It attaches to any ceiling corner and frees up space in your child's bedroom or playroom.

Time Timer

The *Time Timer* allows you to visually understand time perception, i.e., how much time has elapsed or how much is left. You can order it at the following Web site: www.timetimer.com

Travel Receipt Organizer

Do you have trouble keeping track of your receipts? The *Travel Receipt Organizer* is a must have for any car, van, RV, or truck. It has five deep pockets that conveniently store anything from membership cards and receipts to sunglasses. It includes a mileage tracker, pen, and notepad. The top folds down and secures safely with Velcro to keep loose papers from falling out.

* *Watch Minder*

One of the more popular items for folks with AD/HD, the *Watch Minder* is a watch that uses a vibrating system to help you remember tasks. It's great for reminding you when to take your meds. You can order one at the Web site:

www.watchminder.com (Please mention you heard about it here!).

* *Wooden Letter File Organizer*

Pay your bills on time with the *Wooden Letter File Organizer*. It helps you organize your mail/bills by date so that you can get greetings and bills out on time! 31 slots have numbers for each day of the month; just slip the envelopes into the dated slots. Two drawers for pens, stamps, etc. are included.

Sensory Products

* *Bean Bag Chairs*

OTs (occupational therapists) often suggest *Bean Bag Chairs* to place enough pressure on your body to calm yourself down. It's a great way to read comfortably or to just relax.

* *Bed Tent*

When my AD/HD daughter was very young, I couldn't get her to stay in her bed. How did I solve the problem? With a *Bed Tent*. Your child will find the enclosure comforting, allowing him/her to calm down enough to fall asleep.

* *Crystal Spirit Table Top Fountain*

Who can resist the calming sound of water flowing over rocks? Take nature inside and relax with the *Crystal Spirit Table Top Fountain*. The water sounds are incredibly soothing.

*Flannel Socks

If your feet are always cold, winter or summer, try deliciously soft flannel socks. They come in a variety of patterns.

* *Hammock Chair*

    A great way to calm yourself- or your child- is by relaxing in the *Hammock Chair*. It can be installed in a doorway so that it's available year round.

* *Hug00 Comfort Pillow*

    Sometimes we just need a hug to feel better. The *Hug00 Comfort Pillow* is filled with thousands of little micro polystyrene "powder" beads. Remember how good it felt to hug your doll when you were a youngster? Hug away—you'll feel better!

* *Island Melody Wind Chime*

    There's nothing more soothing to the senses than the soft sounds of a chime as the wind gently creates beautiful tones. Check out the *Island Melody Wind Chime*.

Plane Quiet Headphones

    At work or at home, if you really need to block out noise so you can concentrate or relax, the *Plane Quiet Headphones* will do the trick.

Seamless Socks

    Do you hate the feel of seams in your socks? Try *Seamless Socks*! They come in nine colors.

* *Sound Soother*

    The *Sound Soother* offers 20 different soothing environmental sounds to block out noise. Many find it helpful to lull themselves or their child to sleep.

Tag-less T Shirts

> *Tag-less T Shirts* keep cotton next your skin at all times. Women can wear these under their sweaters or for casual wear. They come in various colors and sizes. Great for the AD/HD men and children in their lives, too.

Fidgets

* *Finger Fidgets*

> This product is one I'd never seen before. *Finger Fidgets* offers tactile, visual, and auditory stimulation for those needing sensory stimulation. It has plastic, color-coded, mesh sleeves, containing wood, foam, and chime balls.

Heart Squeeze

> The *Heart Squeeze* is soft, fun, and small enough to take anywhere. It automatically returns to its original shape.

* *Hop Ball*

> Does your child need to move? Don't have time to take him or her to the park for a good workout? Try a *Hop Ball!* They come in three sizes and allow your kids to bounce while holding on to its handle. A great release for hyperactivity while getting a good work out.

* *Klixx*

> *Klixx* are toys made of durable plastic that can be twisted and clicked into an endless variety of shapes! I love *Klixx* because they help during

anxious moments. I used to fidget with this on plane trips, but they work great at the office or in school.

* *Koosh Ball*

The infamous *Koosh Ball* is still a great way to keep those busy hands occupied while working or studying.

* *Mini Trampoline*

Many adults (and kids) with AD/HD report that they can concentrate best while moving. The *Mini Trampoline* is a great way to get your creative juices flowing and expel pent up energy, all while getting a good workout.

* *Rock N Fold Chair*

Is your child hyperactive? Can't get him/her to sit still long enough to finish the homework? Try the *Rock N Fold Chair* and watch your child settle down through movement.

* *Silly Putty*

Remember *Silly Putty*? This is small enough to keep you calm and attentive without anyone even noticing. Not just for kids anymore!

* *Zen Garden*

You've had a long hard day, and all you want to do is zone out and relax. The *Zen Garden* is a tiny personal landscape filled with sand that you can rake while clearing your thoughts and calming your brain.

Products to Simplify Your Life

*Heat-resistant Glove

> Stop burning your hands! This *Heat-resistant Glove* withstands temperatures up to 480 degrees. Now go bake those cookies without hurting yourself!

* iRobot Roomba Robot Vacuum

> Let's face it. Cleaning the house is no picnic. But it can be fun if you have an *iRobot Roomba Robot Vacuum*. Turn on the switch and let it vacuum the house for you.

* Lightweight Poncho/Slicker

> Do you find yourself always getting stuck in a rainstorm without an umbrella or raincoat? The *Lightweight Poncho/Slicker* is so inexpensive and portable that you can buy three per family member. Keep one in the car, one at work or at school, and one at home. No more wet hair or clothes!

* Night Writer Pen

> Your mind is full of ideas, and you can't fall asleep. You don't want to forget what's spinning through your tireless brain, but you also don't want to wake up your partner to write it down before you forget. The *Night Writer Pen* solves that for you. It lights up in the dark!

* Pill Organizer

> If you travel a lot (or a little), you probably get

overwhelmed with all the medications you need to pack, especially if more than one family member takes meds. This handy *Pill Organizer* is a compact wallet with Velcro closures to hold little plastic pill holders.

* *Plant Waterer*

Do you love plants but inadvertently kill them because you forget to water them? The *Plant Waterer* takes the worry out of watering by doing it for you.

* *Rowenta Steam and Press*

One of my favorites is a hand steamer. When I iron, I end up adding more wrinkles, not getting rid of them! The handy *Rowenta Steam and Press* goes with me everywhere.

* *Stay Organized Purse*

The *Stay Organized Purse* has everything you need to be just that: organized! Lots of pockets and compartments to hold all your stuff.

Tip Table Card

When math is a struggle, as it is for many of us, AD/HD or not, then figuring out tips while rushing out of a restaurant or cab can cause one to get even more overwhelmed. This handy little *Tip Table Card* helps you to figure out 10 and 15% tips in just seconds. I use mine all the time. Order yours at the following Web site: www.puffins.com (search for "tip:" *Tip Table Cards*).

* Wrinkle Free Travel Dress

> Don't know what to pack? Or what to wear when you get there? The *Wrinkle Free Travel Dress* solves your travel problems. It can be dressed up with jewelry or worn alone for more casual events.

Software Products for Organization

* ADD Audio Coach

> The *ADD Audio Coach* is a step-by-step coaching system designed specifically to guide and empower adults with ADD to create control, balance, and confidence within their lives. The program includes a 120+ page workbook and a three audio CD set. Areas covered: time management, home organization, personal finances, and project management.

ADD Planner

> *ADD Planner* helps you get to places on time, stay on track at work, plan tasks, and make long-term plans. You can order it at the following Web site: www.addplanner.com

* Christmas Holiday Planner

> End holiday stress, frustration, and chaos with the *Christmas Holiday Planner.* Between holiday card writing, gift giving, decorating, family traditions, baking, and everything else, it's no wonder you're stressed! This software program is chock-full of holiday forms, checklists, logs, and information sheets to help you keep your thoughts and lists organized for a stress-free, joyous, and peaceful Christmas.

* Easy Organizer

Easy Organizer: the easiest way to organize every bit of information in your life! Includes tons of easy to use forms, checklists, logs, and information sheets for important family information, goals, planning, personal growth, home maintenance, cleaning, inventory, gardening, home office, computer, vacations, and more!

eVentSherpa

eVentSherpa helps you organize your busy life! Keep track of events occurring in your home city, your industry, or within your office or social network. You can order it at the following Web site: www.eventsherpa.com
Note: *eVentSherpa™ Lite* is a free version with fewer features. It is a network scheduling tool that allows you to organize your own schedule and subscribe to syndicated event feeds delivered from Web sites around the world. Find it at the following address: www.eventsherpa.com/home/lite.html

GoalPro

Yahoo! Calendar's *GoalPro* is a goal-setting, success-management system with a calendar, journal, scratch pad, reminder system, and more. You can find it at the following Web site: www.goalpro.com

HandyShopper **FREE**!

HandyShopper is a great shopping list tool. Also great for travel packing lists and calorie counting. For Palm OS. You can find it at the following Web site: www.freewarepalm.com/database/handyshopper-english.shtml

Inspiration

Inspiration is a program that lets you develop ideas and organize thinking using diagrams and outlines. Great for students, too. You can order it at the following Web site: www.inspiration.com

Life Balance

Life Balance is a time and task management program that helps you focus on what's really important to you and actively balance the often conflicting demands of career and personal life. *Life Balance* emphasizes the intrinsic importance that you've assigned to your projects and life goals, rather than arbitrarily filling every slot in your calendar. This helps you to spend your time and energy on what matters to you the most. You can be self-directed and know that you are working toward long-term goals while still managing your day to day routine. Also available for PDAs. For more info, visit their Web site at www.llamagraphics.com

* My Budget Planner

Take five minutes a day to budget with *My Budget Planner.* Easy to use, it has versions for kids and teens, too.

PlanPlus

PlanPlus for planning and scheduling in Outlook or for Windows XP. You can find it at the following Web site: www.franklincovey.com/planplus/

RoboForm **FREE!**

Can't remember passwords to access various Web sites? *RoboForm* saves them for you and automatically fills in the forms with your password and any other information you ask of it. You can find it at the following Web site: www.roboform.com/

Student Life

Inexpensive *Student Life* helps you organize every aspect of your college experience. Features: class scheduler, homework and test organizer, contact manager, social activities organizer, reminder manager, degree tracker. You can order it at the following Web site: www.tesorosoft.com/ studentlife.htm

* Taming the Paper Tiger

Do you hate filing? Try *Taming the Paper Tiger*, a powerful filing system that uses the power of your computer to help you get organized and stay organized.

Thought Manager Organizer for Mothers

Thought Manager Organizer for Mothers has over 40 lists and organizers. It includes shopping tools, birthday and trip planning ideas, reference material, home management guides, and more. It lets you create your own lists and organizers easily. The Windows Desktop version includes Palm OS software and synchronization software. You can find it at the following Web site: www.handshigh.com

Time and Chaos

Time and Chaos is contact manager software for Windows users. It organizes your telephone book of contacts and clients and improves your time management capabilities with its appointment calendar and to do list tasks that show you exactly what needs to be done today. If you are on a network, *Time and Chaos* allows you to share your data with everyone in your network with no expensive server add-on required. You can order it at the following Web site: www.chaossoftware.com/

To-Do List **FREE!**

To-Do List is a little software program that is like having a sticky note on your computer desktop. All you have to do is type in your to-do list for the day, check them off when you're done, and you're in good shape for the day. You can find it at the following Web site: www.fp.futuresights.com/ ~angstrom/todolist.html

Parenting Products

* *Job Juggler Chore Chart*

The *Job Juggler Chore Chart* has 135 blank job cards to help you teach your child to become responsible with household chores.

* *Ready Check Go! Picture Check List*

Ready Check Go! Picture Check List shows children, through pictures, what they need to do to get ready in the morning.

* *Better Behavior Wheel*

The *Better Behavior Wheel* has a spinner that lands

on one of eight different consequences, like listening to dad's favorite music or vacuuming the kitchen floor.

Parent Coaching Cards

Parent Coaching Cards were developed by psychologist Dr. Steven Richfield. They are a set of twenty 4" x 6" coated cards with a full-color illustration on one side and a kid-friendly, coping message on the other. Each card depicts a social or emotional skill in language that is easily understood by children from third grade and up. Available at www.parentcoachcards.com

Gift Products
(Help You Save Face When It's Down to the Wire)
*David's Cookies

For the cookie lover, consider *David's Cookies*. Available at: www.davidscookies.com

*1-800-Flowers

One phone call and you're off the hook. Call *1-800-Flowers* or order through my Web site at www.myADDstore (under last minute gifts).

*Popcorn Factory

Want something fun to send? Give large tins of popcorn! They also have other treats and gifts. Available at: www.thepopcornfactory.com

*Tree Givers

Looking for something more unusual? Plant a tree in someone's honor with *Tree Givers*! You can order a tree through the following Web site:

www.treegivers.com . Added bonus: they offer templates if you can't think of words to add to your note.

References

Barkley R., (1995). *Taking charge of AD/HD*. New York: Guilford Press.

Fellman, W. (2000). *Finding a career that works for you.* Plantation, FL: Specialty Press, Inc.

Hallowell, N. and Ratey, N. (1994). *Driven to distraction.* New York: Pantheon Books.

Kelly, K., and Ramundo, P., (1996) *You mean I'm not lazy, stupid or crazy?!* (Reprinted edition). New York: Scribner.

Quinn, P. (Ed.) (1994). *ADD and the college student.* New York: Magination Press.

Solden, S. (1995). *Women with attention deficit disorder.* Grass Valley, CA: Underwood Books.

Weiss, L. (2001). *View from the cliff.* Dallas: Taylor Trade Publishing.

Appendix

Month-of-Meals (MOM) System   324

How to Keep a Kitchen Clean   325

Prioritizing Chart   327

Affirmation List   328

Record Your Own Tips   330

MOM System (Month of Meals)   (#=Day of Month)

1	2	3	4	5	6	7
Pot roast in a bag, mashed potatoes in a bag, can of green beans	Noodles mixed with butter and Parmesan cheese, bagged salad, frozen garlic bread	Deli carry out: cold cuts, onion rolls, potato salad	Breakfast for dinner: scrambled eggs, toast and jam, cut-up fruit	Ready-cooked, whole chicken, 10-minute rice in a bag, canned or frozen peas	Pizza night! Get it delivered.	Smorgasbord: Bring out all leftovers for a buffet-style meal
8	**9**	**10**	**11**	**12**	**13**	**14**
Meatloaf using mix, frozen noodle side dish, frozen broccoli*	Meatloaf sandwiches using leftovers, bagged salad	Canned "hearty" soup, French bread, bagged salad	Hummous, pita bread, can of lentil soup	Carry out Chinese dinner or GO out!	Banquet spaghetti sides, frozen garlic bread, bagged salad**	Frozen finger foods, e.g., mini hotdogs in pastry, spinach pies, mini meatballs, etc.
15	**16**	**17**	**18**	**19**	**20**	**21**
Burgers, canned or frozen corn, bagged salad****	Stouffers' mac and cheese, canned peas, fruit****	Turkey in a bag, mashed potatoes in bag, canned gravy, frozen or canned green beans****	Carry out: kids' choice****	Lunch for dinner: PB & J, tuna, lunch meat sandwiches on special bread or rolls, chips, canned tomato or veg. soup	Meal in a bag with meat already added, bagged salad	Carry-out bagels and flavors of cream cheeses, fruit salad from grocery store
22	**23**	**24**	**25**	**26**	**27**	**28**
Scrambled Eggs Deluxe (add bits of hotdogs, cubed cheese, veggies), canned soup, toast	Prepared pork chops, canned sweetened yams, bagged salad	Pizza night!	Kids' Night to Cook! Suggestions: Sandwiches, fruit salad, and soup*****	Roast beef in a bag, prepared mashed potatoes, canned gravy, bagged salad	Tuna toss, French bread******	Spaghetti with prepared sauce, bagged salad, leftover French bread

* Make two but buy enough ground beef to freeze for future hamburger dinner (see day 15)
** Use 4-5 for dinner portion
*** Use frozen meat from day 6
**** Buy a couple of large boxes
***** Get your children involved in preparing meals
****** See recipe chapter for recipe

How to Keep a Kitchen Clean
by Deborah Lancaster, Sunnyvale, CA

When a kitchen is clean, it's easy to keep it clean. Once it gets dirty, your work is multiplied in order to get it clean. Here are some easy things to do to maintain a clean kitchen:

- Rinse out the sink after you use it. Wash your hands and be sure all the suds go down the drain. Rinse off a dish and be sure the food goes down the drain. Then run the disposal, and it's all taken care of. This takes 10 seconds, and you have a clean sink!

- Wipe off the counter and cutting board after you use them.

- Make a sandwich, do the dishes, chop an onion, and then wipe the counter; it takes about 10 seconds.

- Use kitchen wipes (Clorox, Costco brand) or damp paper towels, then toss.

- Wipe around the stove after you cook.

- Spills, boil overs, bubbling liquids—all of these will deposit food on the stove top. Clean it while it's still warm, and it only takes 10 seconds; wait until it's cold, and it takes longer and looks messy in the meantime. Use the kitchen wipes or paper towels, then toss.

- Clean the floor if you spill something.

- Put the hand towel by the sink so you don't have to drip water across the floor on your way to get it; this water is what makes dirt stick to the floor. If you move a pan from the stove to the dishwasher (*not* the sink!) and it drips, wipe the floor. If you spill your drink on the way out of the kitchen, go back and clean it up. It only takes 5 seconds and prevents the floor from getting even more dirty as things stick to that liquid for the next several days or weeks.

- Use the sponge and dish brush *only* for dishes and the counter, then rinse, squeeze, and replace. Do not wipe the floor with the kitchen sponge; use a kitchen wipe or paper towel for that, then toss it. Wipe the sink and counter with the sponge or clean off the dishes; same for the dish brush. Then rinse, squeeze, and replace the sponge; that leaves it ready for the next person so that they don't have to pick up a sponge full of cold dirty water and bits of old food. *Gross!!*

- Use the hand towel only for your hands; it is not for the counter, the dishes, or the floor. This is the terry cloth one with loops in the fabric.

- Use a dish towel only for dishes; it is not for the counter, your hands, or the floor. This is the cotton towel that is flat (no loops in the fabric).

- Run your dishwasher every night and empty it every morning. That way it's always ready for dirty dishes during the day.

- Wipe appliances before putting them away: mixer, blender, crock pot, food processor, etc.

- Materials you'll need to keep your kitchen clean: kitchen wipes (Clorox, Costco, Lysol brands), sponge, dish brush, paper towels, terry cloth hand towels and flat cotton dish towels.

Prioritizing Chart
by Deborah Lancaster, Sunnyvale, CA

TASK	Important	Urgent	Total
_____	_____	_____	_____
_____	_____	_____	_____
_____	_____	_____	_____
_____	_____	_____	_____

Now rewrite your list in order of priority:

_____ _____

_____ _____

_____ _____

_____ _____

Remember: Not every task can be a "1!" I know it feels that way but think about it a little more. Ask yourself, "What will happen if I don't do this?" This applies to both urgency and importance. Advanced techniques—try these only when you have mastered the basics:

1. Alternate required tasks with fun tasks, matching them by estimated time for completion. This requires great discipline.
2. Use the scale 1-4 (1 is a lot, 4 is not really) to determine how much you want to do a task. Add this number to the total and then rewrite the list.
3. Add a column for estimated time to completion.
4. Time yourself and write down the actual time to completion.

Note: Deborah picked this tip up got at a Discovery Toys convention at least 12 years ago, and though she didn't write it, she does use it and share it at local and national conferences where she presents on the topic of procrastination.

Affirmations
by Linda Anderson, M. A., MCC

- I am organized.
- I like order.
- I like simplicity.
- I like having just enough...and not too much.
- I am changing.
- I am growing.
- I am allowed to make mistakes.
- I am taking action steps.
- I am a thinking person.
- I am a doing person.
- I am a feeling person.
- I am becoming.
- I am responsible.
- I like challenge.
- I invite change.
- I have a mission. I have values. I have purpose.
- I give up that which is not necessary.
- I can say no.
- I keep only that which nurtures and supports me.
- I let go of what I do not need, which holds me back.
- I am safe.
- It gives me great pleasure to organize my things so that when I am looking for something, I know where to find it.
- Day by day, I get better and better at letting papers and old stuff go.
- That which I did not invite into my space, I do not let in.
- My boundaries are clear and strong.

- I do the laundry because it makes me feel good.
- I put things away because I'm taking care of business and living my life.
- I sort mail and pay bills; it makes me feel good to be clear, responsible, and free of paper clutter.
- I put things away after using them because it feels good to follow through.
- I buy only what I need and trust that there will always be enough.
- I throw away things that take up my space. I give away things I don't need. I enjoy what I have left.
- I enjoy openness and space around me in which to create whatever I choose to create.
- I am a creative being.
- It gives me great pleasure to organize things so that I can enjoy them and use them to their fullest.
- I seek balance in my life.
- I take the time to breathe.
- I take the time to stop and look around me.
- I take the time to enjoy the moment.
- As I give up the stuff I've kept around me, I discover more of who I am.
- I am a good and worthy person.

Record Your Own Tips

Index

Symbols

504 Plan, 131

A

AD/HD Information and Support
 Services ADDISS (UK),
 295, 300
AD/HD News, 295
ADA Information Line (U.S.
 Dept. of Justice), 300
ADD at About.com, 295
ADD Coach Academy, 302
ADD Consults, 295, 299
ADD Consults Coach Directory,
 302
ADD Forums, 295
ADD International Professionals,
 297
ADD Professionals, 297
ADD Resources, 295, 300
ADD Warehouse, 298
ADDers.org, 295
ADDitional News, 255, 297
ADDitude Magazine, 297
ADDmirableWomen, 294
ADDvance, 294
ADDvisor, 297
All Kinds of Minds, 303
Amen, Daniel, 301
American Coaching Association,
 302
Anderson, Linda, 193–195
ATTENTION , 298
Attention Deficit Disorder
 Association (ADDA),
 295, 300
Attention Research Update, 298

B

Barkley, Russell, 132, 321

C

Children and Adults with Atten-
 tion-deficit/Hyperactivity
 Disorder, 296, 300
Conveniencenet.com, 302

D

Debtors Anonymous, 141

E

Eddy, Cindy, 211
Equal Employment Opportunity
 Commission, 300

F

Fellman, Wilma, 88, 244–
 246, 321
FOCUS, 298

G

Get Organized Now!, 302
Giwerc, David, 195, 251-253
Goldstein, Sam, 301
Granger, Melody, 211–212

H

Hallowell, Edward, 2, 227–
 228, 301, 321
Hartmann, Thom, 230–232, 302

Household chores tips,
  cleaning and decluttering, 51–54
  dishes, 54–56
  errands, 56–57
  laundry, 47–51
Humorous side,
  kitchen chaos, 178–180
  quotes from impatient patients, 183–191
  stories to tickle the funny bone, 176–178
  you know you have AD/HD when, 163–176
Hypersensitivity, 10, 12

I

Individual Education Plan (IEP), 131

J

Jaksa, Peter, 246–249, 302
Job Accommodation Network, 300, 303
Job Applicants and the Americans with Disabilities, 303
Johnson, Mary Jane, 199–201

K

Kelly, Kate, 3, 234–237, 302, 321
Koretsky, Jennifer, 201–203

L

LD Online, 296
Learning Disability Association of America (LDA), 301
List Organizer, 302

Living with ADD, 296

M

Mahia, Lee, 212–213
Making decisions, 12
Managing finances tips,
  paying bills, 136–137
  saving money, 139–141
Marlowe, Alita, 213–214
Martin, Reed, 132, 299, 303
McConlogue, Kerch, 203–207
McCurdy, Sheila, 214–215
Meal planning, 12
Meals and entertaining tips,
  cooking, 32–37
  entertaining at home, 37–45
  grocery shopping, 29–32
  meal planning 37–43
Memory tips, 12
  capturing ideas, 143–145
  keeping track of things, 145–146
  miscellaneous tips, 147–148
  names, 149–151
  physiology of memory, 146–147
  reminders, 151–152
  timers, 152–153
Messies Anonymous, 300
Mind Tools, 303
Mitchell, Ginger, 215–217
Mitchell, Jennifer 215–217
myADD Store, 296
myADHD.com, 296

N

National Association for Professional Organizers, 301, 302
National Center for Gender Issues

and AD/HD, 294, 301
National Institute of Mental
 Health (NIMH) AD/HD,
 296
National Resource Center for AD/
 HD, 297
National Study Group on the
 Chronically Disorganiz
 301, 303

O

Online Organizing.com, 303
Optimal Functioning Institute,
 302
Organize Tips, 303
Organized-Mom, 303
Organizing tips,
 closets and shelves, 19–20
 general, 26–28
 kids and their clutter, 20–21
 kitchen area, 15–18
 paper, 21–25

P

Paige, Kris, 206–207
Parenting, 12
Parenting and family tips,
 behavior and discipline, 119–
 123
 chores, 126–127
 family time and personal time,
 127
 minimizing distractions, 124–
 126
 sleep, 124
 traveling with kids, 123–124
Personal tips,
 clothes shopping and dressing,
 62–65

health, 65–67
hypersensitivities, 67
leisure time, 76–77
miscellaneous, 74–75
sleep, 73
travel, 75–76
President's Committee on
 Employment of People with
 Disabilities, 301

Q

Quinn, Patricia, 232–234, 321

R

Ramundo, Peggy, 3, 321
Ratey, John, 2, 302, 321
Ratey, Nancy, 208–210, 241–
 244, 302
Recipes, 255–286
Relationships, 11
Relationships and social skills
 tips,
 general advice, 111–112
 support, 112–113
Resources,
 media, websites, newsletters,
 mailing lists, magaz 294
 products, 304–320
 support, 299
 websites of AD/HD experts,
 301
Richards, Linda, 217–218
Richardson, Wendy, 302
Robin, Arthur, 249–253

S

Saunders, Ann, 218–219
Schmidt, Rebecca, 219–220

Schwab Learning Foundation, 297

Seidler, Cyndi, 220–221

Sequencing, 13

Sidetracked Home Executives, 303

Solden, Sari, 5, 11, 228–230, 294, 302, 321

Sort-It, 303

Study strategies, 81–85

T

Technology tips,
Internet, 159–162
Palm Pilot uses, 155–159, 217–218

The AD/HD Report, 298

Time and data management tips,
capturing ideas, 101–103
data management, 98–99
planners, 99–101
time management, 105–109
timers, 104–105

Tips from AD/HD experts, 225–253

Tips from professional coaches, 193–211

Tips from professional organizers, 211–223

U

U.S. Department of Education Regional of People wi 301

U.S. Equal Employment Opportunity Commission, 303

Umansky, Peggy, 221–222

W

Weiss, Lynn, 237–241, 321

White del Rosso, Kristin, 222–223

Workplace tips,
careers, 87–88
clutter, 94
general, 94–95
minimizing distractions, 91–93
organizing tasks, 90
scheduling, 93

Wright, Peter 132

Wright's Law, 303